THE BIG BOOK OF
KETO
DIET
COOKING

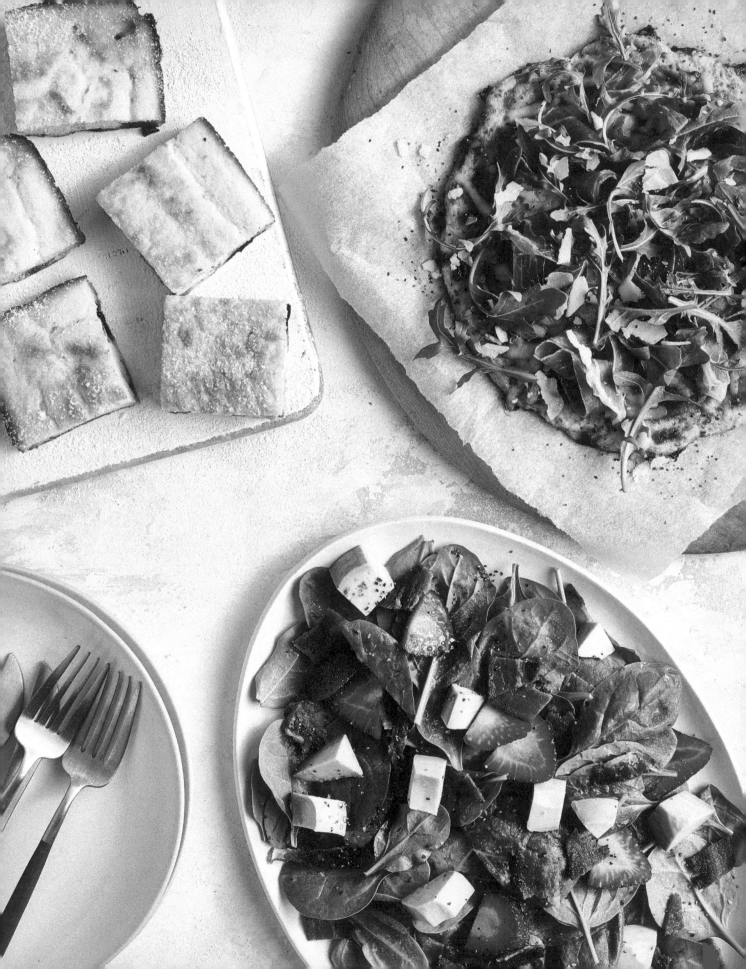

THE BIG BOOK OF
KETO DIET
COOKING

200 Everyday Recipes and Easy 2-Week Meal
Plans for a Healthy Keto Lifestyle

JEN FISCH

Photography by Hélène Dujardin

ROCKRIDGE
PRESS

Designer: Katy Brown
Editor: Pippa White
Production Editor: Andrew Yackira
Photography © Hélène Dujardin, 2018; styling by Tami Hardeman
Author photo © Suzanne Strong

Cover: Pan-Seared T-Bone Steak with Herby Butter, page 182

ISBN: Print 978-1-93975-426-4 | eBook 978-1-93975-427-1

R1

*To my Kaia Bear,
my daughter and
Chief Taste Tester*

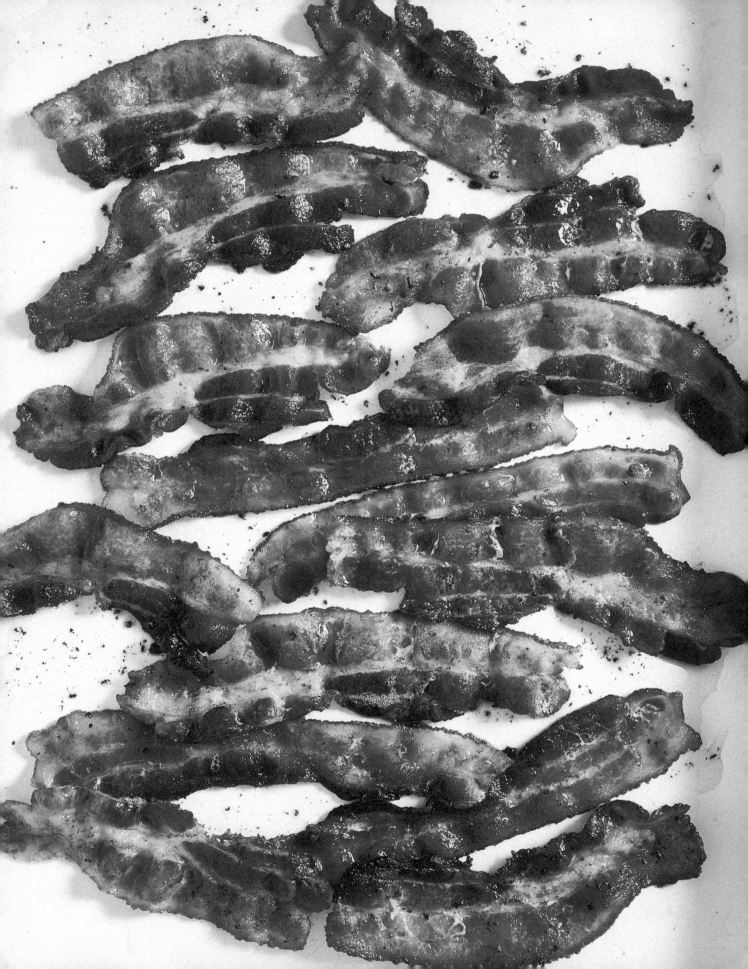

CONTENTS

FOREWORD

WHEN JEN ASKED ME to write the foreword of her book, it was the easiest "yes" I've given in a long time.

I started my keto journey in February of 2017. In my early stages of online research, Jen's Instagram account @KetoInTheCity_ was the very first one I found. Jen immediately captured my attention. Not only was she beautiful and confident, but her content was rich and so easy to understand. Keto can be tricky. There are a million different ways to approach a keto lifestyle, and it can become overwhelming fast. When I found Jen's account, I felt like I had finally found some guidance. Her recipes were simple, they didn't use any strange ingredients that deterred me from trying out different dishes, and she always made keto seem like something I could realistically do for life.

I learned from Jen that a ketogenic diet doesn't have to be difficult or fussy, and I am still inspired by her daily. In fact, she even motivated me to start my very own keto Instagram account! I wanted to show the world that keto can be done in the most basic form, and you don't need to overcomplicate it. I learned the bedrock of the keto diet from Jen, and I am so grateful to her.

I was fortunate enough to be able to meet Jen in real life in June of this year. You would think that we would've done something super exciting involving delicious keto food, but nope! We sat on the couch and talked for hours about how this way of eating has completely changed us for the better. We swapped success stories, busy mom stories, and everything in between. Jen has a true passion for all things keto and is an incredibly hard worker. You can feel her love for the keto lifestyle in these recipes.

I so badly wish that this book had been around when I first started my journey. This cookbook lays it all out in such a simple form. In these pages, Jen offers an intro to what keto is, a chart of keto-friendly foods to eat/avoid, shopping lists, meal plans, and best of all, tons of EASY recipes! This will be your go-to keto bible, and I am excited for you to be inspired by Jen, just like I have been.

I am so proud of her accomplishments and am still a bit starstruck that she has asked me to be a part of this book. After all, she has been my keto guru. I can't wait for you to dive in and take advantage of the knowledge she provides here. You're gonna love it!

—Julie Smith, @KetoMadeSimple

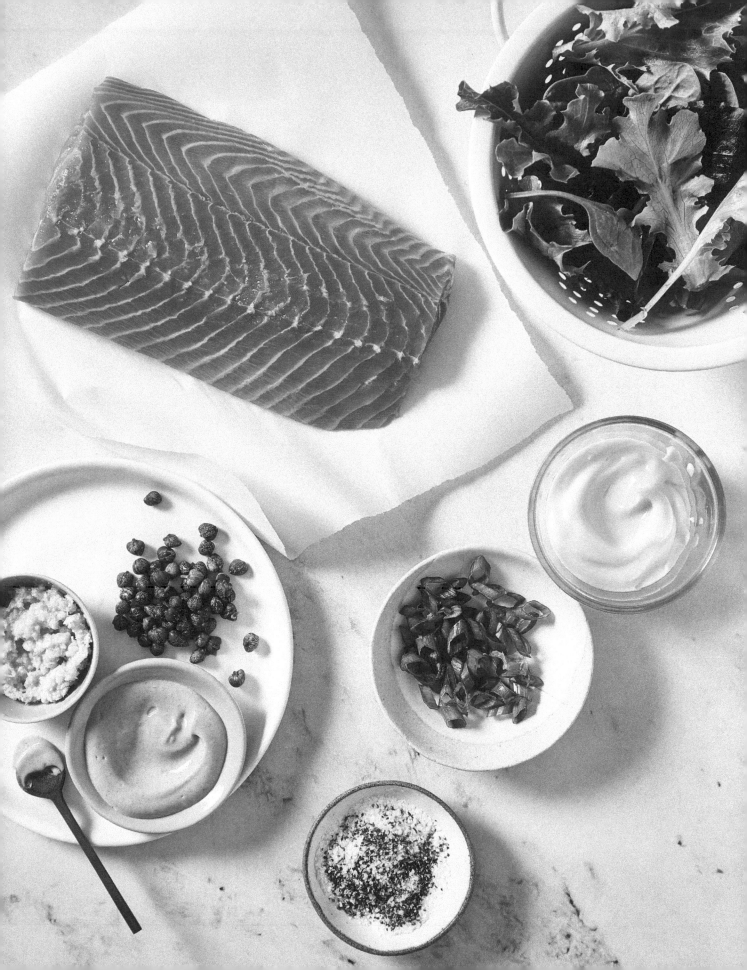

INTRODUCTION

I STARTED FOLLOWING a ketogenic lifestyle because I was searching for a way of eating that would help relieve some of the inflammation I experience from my two autoimmune disorders, psoriatic arthritis and psoriasis. I have been fighting these diseases for about 20 years, and during that time I have learned that eating an anti-inflammatory diet can be a great tool. Food alone isn't going to save my joints from the damaging effects of psoriatic arthritis, but it is important to me that I know I'm doing everything I can to complement the treatment set forth by my doctors.

Weight loss was also an important motivator for me beginning keto. Over the last two years of following a ketogenic diet, I have lost 30 pounds. Some people will lose weight faster than that—some lose 30 pounds within a few months of starting keto, as everyone's body is different. What I know is that I feel so much better than I did a couple of years ago, and that is hugely important to me. As a single working mom, I need to have a ton of energy to survive the daily grind, and keto does that for me. It also helps me sleep like a baby at night, which is so important for all of us in these sleep-deprived times.

I started cooking more frequently about 10 years ago, mainly so that I could have a stress-relieving creative outlet after work. I'm not a chef or a nutritionist. I am just a tired (and hungry) mom who wanted to make quick, healthy meals for my daughter and myself. Since I began cooking more, I've come to really enjoy it. My intention with this book is to help you make cooking one of the best parts of your day, like it is with mine.

I also want to help you learn how the ketogenic diet can be an important tool in your life. Switching to a new way of eating is always a bit of an adjustment, but I promise to make it as simple (and delicious) as possible! Whether you have turned to keto for weight loss, for healing, or for both, I will show you how you can be successful using familiar flavors.

I often hear people say that eating keto must be expensive or super overwhelming. I am here to tell you it is not. Keto can be easy to prepare, unfussy, and just plain yummy. You don't need recipes with a list of 30 ingredients or a million steps. If you have my first book, *The Easy 5-Ingredient Ketogenic Diet Cookbook*, then you know that amazing meals can be created with just a few ingredients. With keto, you will get to simplify your pantry and focus on cooking with delicious healthy fats and fresh ingredients.

I've titled this book *The Big Book of Ketogenic Diet Cooking* because I wanted to give you an all-in-one resource that can be your bible of ketogenic diet cooking. It features tons of recipe ideas for new and seasoned keto-ers so that you never run out of things to cook.

Here you will find simple recipes that deliver great flavor and use ingredients you can find in any grocery store. I happen to love wandering aimlessly down the aisles of a grocery store (it is oddly therapeutic for me), but you don't have to do that for these recipes! Each recipe has easy-to-find ingredients, so you can spend your free time wandering around somewhere else. As we dive into the book, I will give you a brief overview of the principles of the ketogenic diet, but this book is focused on the recipes. (See the Resources section at the back of the book to learn more about the science behind keto eating.) The recipes in this book are designed for people who are looking to stay within 20 to 50 net carbs per day. Under each recipe you will see the macro breakdown as a quick and easy tool to track your carb intake.

Being successful on keto or any healthy eating plan is determined by two main factors:

1. How satisfied are you?

2. How practical is this way of eating for your everyday life?

The recipes in this book keep these factors in mind. Eating a diet full of healthy fats will leave you feeling satisfied, and the sheer number of recipes will show you that you don't have to miss any foods on keto—instead you just need to keto-fy those carb-filled comfort foods you used to eat. I will show you how to do that in your everyday life with simple, easy-to-follow recipes. I have also included three two-week meal plans in this book—which you can use as guides. The meal plans take the guesswork out of choosing recipes and designing each day of eating.

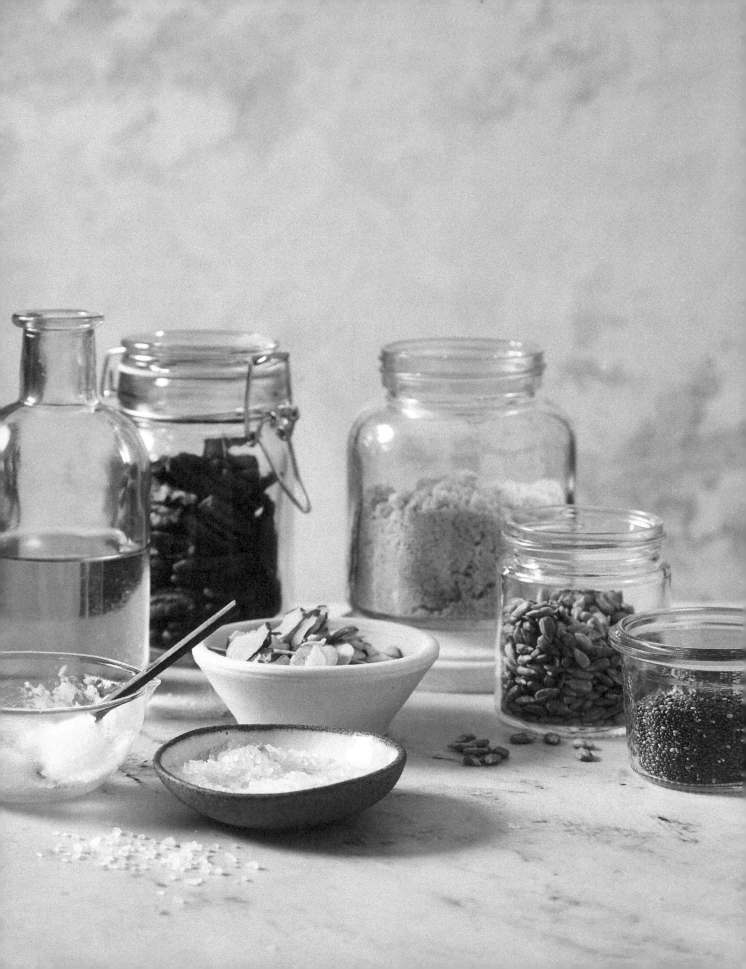

KETOGENIC DIET COOKING

CHAPTER ONE

One of the first things you'll want to do to get ready for all of the keto cooking that's about to happen is to prep your pantry and give your kitchen a keto makeover. But first, let's dive into the basics of eating keto. Here I will introduce you to the ins and outs of eating keto, help you put together your new and improved keto pantry, and show you everything you need to do to get started on this exciting new culinary journey.

EATING KETO

The ketogenic diet is a high-fat, moderate-protein, and low-carb diet. By drastically restricting the amount of carbs and sugar you eat, your body burns its own fat (ketones) instead of glucose. This happens because your liver converts fat into fatty acids, and the ketone bodies pass into your brain and replace glucose as your energy source. This is known as ketosis, and it is the goal of the ketogenic diet.

HIGH FAT

The standard keto diet is typically made up of about 70 percent healthy fats. When I first started keto, I had no problem restricting carbs, but it took some real effort to get my fat levels high enough. The fats are what makes keto fun and sustainable for the long term. Bacon, avocado, egg yolks, salmon, and cream cheese are all on the keto menu! Getting high ratios of fats in every meal is important because it helps you feel full and satiated. Once you are fat-adapted, you will find your-self needing to eat less frequently thanks to the high levels of fat you are consuming.

Common sources of fat in keto are full-fat dairy, fatty cuts of meat and fish, grass-fed butter, and high-quality oils.

MODERATE PROTEIN

The protein levels of keto are an important differentiator in comparison to other low-carb ways of eating. Anyone who has done high-protein, low-carb diets in the past may be familiar with the feeling of always being hangry (hungry + angry) and never feeling full. This doesn't happen on keto because you will keep your protein at a moderate level and raise your intake of fats. If you consume too much protein, it can turn into glucose, so you want to make sure you don't overdo it because it can kick you out of ketosis. A typical keto diet is made up of about 25 percent protein.

Common sources of protein in keto are meat, fish, and eggs.

LOW CARB

By now you know that keto is a low-carb way of eating, and you have probably noticed that we have just 5 percent left to complete 100 percent of the diet. Well, that is where the carbs come in! A standard American diet is somewhere in the 50 to 60 percent range for carbs, so it is a big difference and a major adjustment for your body. Most people following the ketogenic diet consume between 20 and 50 net carbs a day, and this is the suggested amount of carbs to stay in ketosis. Net carbs are calculated by subtracting a food's total fiber from its total carbs. So if 1 cup of broccoli has 6g of carbs and 2g of fiber, the net carb amount is 4g. Additionally, if you are eating something that has sugar alcohols in it, you also subtract that from the total when calculating net carbs. Personally, I aim for 20 grams of net carbs each day. Some people count actual carbs instead of net carbs. It is a personal choice, so choose what works best for you and your goals.

Often we think of carbs as bread and bread-like foods, but carbs can be found in other foods, as well. The most common sources of carbs on a keto diet are vegetables—my favorites are dark leafy greens and cruciferous vegetables like broccoli and cauliflower.

MACRONUTRIENTS

Macronutrients or "macros" are terms that are used widely in information about the ketogenic diet, so let's start with understanding what they are, how you can figure them out, and how to use them.

Essentially, macronutrients are the three components that make up all kinds of food. Our food breaks down into three distinct macronutrients: fat, protein, and carbohydrates. Fat has more calories per gram than protein and carbs, making it the most energy-dense macronutrient. This is important because while you're on the keto diet, you will find you will not need to eat as much food, because so much of the food you will be eating will be full of fats.

To figure out what your ideal macros are, you can use keto macro calculators online. I have one on my website, ketointhecity.com, and you can find them on other keto websites as well. You will enter your activity level, gender, size, and goals, and it will recommend personalized suggested daily macros for your body. You can then take those macros and set your preferences in an app like Carb Manager or MyFitnessPal. Then as you track your food, it will show you the macronutrient ratios you are hitting. I found this to be very helpful when I began keto.

Some people track their macros and some people don't. It's a decision that you'll make on your own, but I find it helpful to at least calculate the macros so you can have a target in mind and eat more consciously.

All Fats Are Not Created Equal

The type of fats you eat is very important. Keto is focused on the good fats. Fats are important as a source of energy and also for keeping you full and satisfied. Eating a mix of healthy fats can help raise your levels of "good" cholesterol (HDL) while lowering the "bad" (LDL). The good fats you want to include on a keto diet include:

- Monounsaturated fats: avocados, olives, macadamia nuts

- Saturated fats: grass-fed butter, meats, ghee, coconut oil

- Polyunsaturated omega-3s: salmon, sardines, chia seeds, walnuts

- Medium-chain triglycerides (also known as MCTs): coconut oil, dairy products, MCT oil

The bad fats are refined oils like corn, vegetable, and canola oils. Artificial trans fats like margarine and Crisco are also bad fats. It is easy to avoid these low-quality products if you are cooking in your own home and have cleared your pantry, but eating out is another challenge. Fast-food restaurants and other restaurants often use these lower-quality oils, so it is always best to ask.

FLEXIBILITY AND BALANCE

Now that you know your macros, you can plan your day of eating around them. I like to look at my macros as my allowance for the day. Would you rather eat three meals a day or spend the majority of your macros on one big meal? It's genuinely up to you! Keto provides the flexibility to design your own day of eating.

A Note on Cholesterol

A lot of people have questions about keto and cholesterol. I got my cholesterol checked at the beginning of my keto journey, and again every year so that I can compare the results. I am happy to say that my total cholesterol has gone down every year since beginning keto. From 2017 to 2018 alone my total cholesterol reduced by 30 points. There have been studies that show that a ketogenic diet can be an effective way to raise heart-healthy HDL cholesterol. There are lists online for keto-friendly doctors, and I would recommend finding one in your area and consulting with them on the best tests to get periodically. There are also books available focused just on keto and cholesterol.

The majority of the time I start my day with a Fatty Latte (page 82), then have a large lunch and a smaller dinner. Two meals a day works well for me, and the fatty coffee in the morning keeps me full enough to wait until lunch. The most important thing is that you listen to your body. If you are hungry, then eat! Similarly, if you are not hungry, don't force a meal on yourself just to hit macros. One of my favorite parts about keto is that I have truly begun to listen to my body's needs, which can differ from day to day or week to week. The recipes in this book provide a wide variety of options so you can choose recipes that work with your daily goals.

THE CHOOSE AND LOSE LISTS

Here are the basic foods you can use in your everyday cooking along with the foods you will want to cross off your grocery list. I believe in buying the highest-quality ingredients you can afford. I know it is expensive to buy grass-fed meats and wild-caught salmon, but ultimately I am doing keto to reduce inflammation in my body, so I want to make sure I am not ingesting unnecessary chemicals and preservatives. Factory-farmed meat and seafood are much lower in nutrients and may contain nasty preservatives and nitrates, which can cause a lot of issues in your body (like inflammation). So do the best you can, and whenever possible buy the highest-quality version of a food that you can find.

FOODS TO CHOOSE

- Grass-fed butter and/or ghee
- Extra-virgin olive oil and/or avocado oil
- Wild-caught seafood
- Grass-fed meats
- Pasture-raised chicken and pork
- Pasture-raised eggs
- Uncured, nitrate-free bacon
- Cruciferous vegetables: arugula, bok choy, broccoli, Brussels sprouts, cabbage, cauliflower, collard greens, kale
- Other vegetables: asparagus, celery, cucumbers, peppers, spinach, squash, zucchini
- Full-fat dairy: organic cream cheese, sour cream, heavy whipping cream, cheese
- Full-fat coconut milk and cream
- Nuts: almonds, walnuts, macadamia nuts, pecans
- Seeds: chia seeds, flaxseed, sunflower seeds
- Fatty fruit: avocado, olives
- Berries
- Cacao and sugar-free chocolate
- Sweetener: erythritol, stevia, xylitol
- Pink Himalayan salt
- Drinks: water, sparkling water, coffee, unsweetened tea
- Flour: almond flour, almond meal, coconut flour

FOODS TO LOSE

- Margarine
- Low-quality oils: corn, canola, vegetable, soybean
- Factory-farmed fish
- Processed meats
- Starchy vegetables: potatoes, yams, beans, peas, corn
- Milk
- Higher-carb nuts: pistachios, cashews
- Fruits other than berries
- Dried fruit
- Sugary drinks: juice, energy drinks
- Sugary sweeteners: sugar, agave, honey
- Flour: all-purpose flour, corn flour, rice flour, wheat flour

PANTRY ESSENTIALS

Having the right foods on hand is so important to being successful on keto. It makes cooking so much easier, and there is only a short list of products that I would consider truly essential.

Olive oil or avocado oil: Avocado oil has a higher smoke point and a milder flavor than olive oil. I like to use avocado oil to cook and olive oil for drizzling over dishes like a caprese salad. Avocado oil used to be harder to find, but now it is pretty widely available.

Pink Himalayan salt: I had never bought pink salt until I went keto, and now I am obsessed. Salt is important on keto because you are not eating processed carbs, which are generally loaded with sodium, so you want to make sure you get your salt in and that it is high quality. Pink Himalayan salt has over 84 minerals and trace elements, including important things like calcium, magnesium, copper, and iron. So it is good for you and makes everything taste better! I recommend using pink Himalayan salt for every recipe in this book that requires salt.

Almond flour or almond meal: I use these two interchangeably, as almond flour is just more refined than almond meal. I tend to use almond flour more, but there are certain dishes like Pepperoni and Pepperoncini FatHead Pizza (page 162) where I enjoy the added texture that almond meal provides.

Coconut flour: Coconut and almond flour do not act the same way, so throughout the book you will see that some recipes call for one or the other. I do not recommend switching out one for the other unless you are very experienced in converting these two ingredients.

Coconut milk: I always use canned coconut milk because it has fewer additives than coconut in a carton and has an authentic coconut milk taste. Oftentimes the canned variety has a low-fat option—for keto recipes, you want to use the full-fat option.

Sweetener: You have options when it comes to sweeteners. I tend to use erythritol and stevia the most. Some people have a super-strong preference, so use what you like the best. In my last book I used stevia for the recipes, and in this book I use erythritol. There are many online resources that show conversions across all sweeteners if you would like to substitute. When I use erythritol, I use the Swerve brand because they have granular and confectioner varieties, which is great. I also use Xylitol sometimes, but you should be aware that Xylitol is not safe for animals. I don't have any pets, so it is not an issue in my house, but it may be in yours. Please note that though technically erythritol is a carbohydrate, its effect on blood sugar is a net zero, so it should never be counted as a carbohydrate when calculating macros. For this reason, you'll see that every recipe in the book that includes erythritol has been calculated without factoring it in, and instead has a separate listing for the amount of erythritol in the recipe.

Cacao: Cacao (not to be confused with cocoa!) is the pure form of chocolate as it is harvested from nature. Cacao is not processed with high heat, so it keeps its nutrients, such as magnesium, antioxidants, and iron. I always buy raw cacao to ensure there is no sugar or other ingredients added in. Cacao can be purchased in powder form as well as in nibs, and I always have both on hand.

Sneaky Gluten

Keto is naturally a gluten-free way of eating. If you stick to simple, natural ingredients like meat, fish, vegetables, and full-fat dairy, you won't have to worry about gluten. However, you need to be careful with store-bought ingredients if you are looking to avoid gluten completely. Common products that some people enjoy on keto that often contain gluten include low-carb tortillas, some brands of mayonnaise, egg substitutes, hot dogs, and regular soy sauce. So make sure you check for the "gluten-free" label on products and make sure the majority of your diet is coming from "real foods" and you will be fine!

FRIDGE FAVORITES

Just like a well-stocked pantry, a well-stocked refrigerator can make it easy to whip up a healthy keto meal. I'm not one to eat the same meals over and over again, but there are definitely some key items I always have in my refrigerator no matter what.

Grass-fed butter or ghee: These two are interchangeable in recipes. Personally, I use grass-fed butter, but if you are avoiding dairy, then ghee is a great choice for you. Yes, ghee is made from butter, but it is pure butter fat without the milk solids, which can be inflammatory. So within this book, ghee is considered dairy free. Whether you choose butter or ghee, I highly recommend making sure it is grass-fed. It tastes better and has a better fatty acid ratio.

Eggs: I love the orange yolks from pasture-raised eggs. Pasture-raised eggs have more nutrients than conventionally raised eggs, so buy the highest quality you can afford.

Greens: I typically always have fresh spinach on hand. I throw it in everything from eggs to pasta to smoothies. Spinach is a great source of potassium and magnesium, which are very useful in managing your electrolytes on keto.

Cauliflower and cauliflower rice: I love cauliflower and always have a head or fresh precut florets on hand. When I call for riced cauliflower throughout this book, I mean that it is processed into tiny pieces about the size of rice. You can easily make cauliflower rice in a food processor. Additionally, many grocery stores have it already cut to size and packaged in the produce section.

Low-carb vegetables: Broccoli, cucumbers, and celery.

Low-carb fruits: Avocado, grape tomatoes, and berries.

Heavy whipping cream or full-fat coconut milk: I like to buy organic, and I alternate between heavy cream and canned coconut milk, depending on the recipe.

Bacon: You will almost never find my refrigerator without bacon unless I just devoured the last of it. Look for uncured bacon without nitrates. I also love to buy bacon ends and pieces, which are less expensive and work great for recipes where you cut up or crumble the bacon anyway.

Pepperoncini, capers, pickles, and olives: If I want quick and easy ways to add a punch of flavor to different dishes, I always go for one of these four briny, delicious items. I love them all equally and use them frequently on keto-friendly pizzas, roasted cauliflower, and more.

Shirataki noodles: I always have these carb-free and calorie-free noodles on hand for use in a variety of "pasta" shapes. I use the Miracle Noodle brand because they offer shapes like fettuccine, angel hair, and ziti (my favorite)! Zoodles (zucchini noodles) are also a good keto noodle replacement. There's some debate as to whether these noodles are paleo. Within this book, I consider them to be paleo friendly.

Cheese: I love cheese and usually have a variety in my refrigerator. A lot of people say not to buy the preshredded cheese on keto because it often has added potato starch that keeps it from sticking together, but I do buy it because my sore and arthritic hands do not enjoy grating cheese.

Condiments: Mayonnaise, Sriracha, and mustard. I purchase avocado oil–based mayo that is made with cage-free eggs. I find this is much higher quality than standard mayo, especially in terms of the oils.

Sugar-free dark chocolate: This is great to have on hand when you want something sweet. I love the ChocZero brand.

Meat, poultry, and seafood: I tend to make dishes with a lot of the same proteins over and over again. Wild-caught salmon, grass-fed ground beef, pork chops, and organic chicken drumsticks, thighs, or breasts are on my regular shopping list.

Sweeteners on a Keto Diet

As I mentioned in the Pantry Essentials on page 5, I use erythritol and stevia the most. The macros in this book are calculated using erythritol. Erythritol is a sugar alcohol that does not spike blood sugar and has a glycemic index of zero. Erythritol is absorbed by the small intestine and then 90 percent is eliminated by the body, so it is never metabolized. So while 1 teaspoon of erythritol has 4g of carbs, when calculating, you subtract 4g of the sugar alcohols, leaving you with zero net carbs. Because erythritol does not affect blood sugar, the carbohydrates are considered nonimpact.

Note: All recipes in this book that include a sweetener use erythritol for nutrition calculations.

ESSENTIAL EQUIPMENT

Food processor: I use a small one since I am generally just cooking for my daughter and myself. It was inexpensive and works great. I don't have a good blender or bullet, so I use my food processor for so many things!

Mixer or hand mixer: I have a hand mixer that was also inexpensive, but if you have a nice big countertop model, that works great too.

Skillet: A nice-size skillet will work for so many dishes. I know a lot of people love cast iron skillets, but I don't like holding a pan that heavy (due to my arthritis), so I stick with a regular skillet.

Casserole: I have several different sizes of casserole dishes, but since I generally cook for just two people, I use the small ones the most. You will get a lot of use out of a 9-by-9-inch pan.

Baking sheet: A large baking sheet is great for roasting veggies and much more.

Silicone baking mat: I like to use my silicone baking mat with my baking sheet. It's easy to wash and to reuse, but you can use parchment paper if you'd prefer.

Slow cooker: I love my slow cooker, even though it's all banged up and as basic as they come. You don't need a fancy one as long as it will cook on low and high. Some pressure cookers also have slow cooker settings.

Ramekins or muffin tin: These are great for making individual servings of desserts and keto breads, but also good for quick egg dishes.

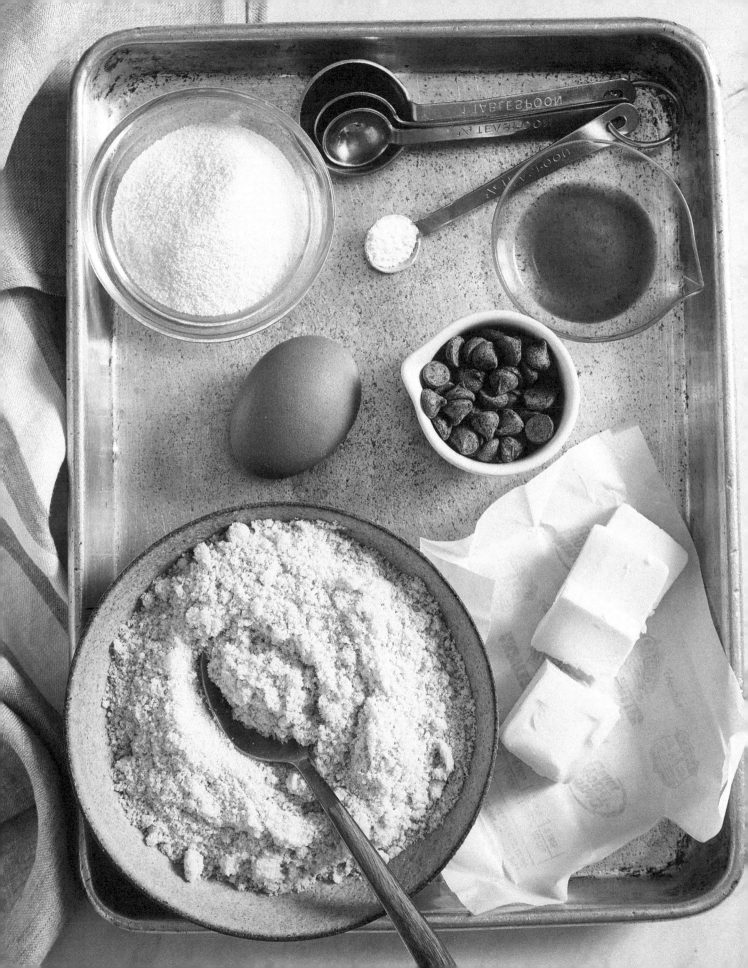

High-Carb Comfort Foods Made Keto

HIGH-CARB COMFORT FOOD	SERVING SIZE	NET CARBS	KETO-FRIENDLY ALTERNATIVE	SERVING SIZE	NET CARBS
Pasta	1 cup	41g	Shirataki noodles or Zoodles	1 cup 1 cup	<1g 4g
Pepperoni Pizza	2 slices	44g	Pepperoni FatHead Pizza or Skillet Pizza	2 slices 1 pizza	5.5g 2g
Cheesecake	1 slice	20g	Cheesecake Bar	1 bar	7g
Mashed Potatoes	1 cup	32g	Mashed Cauliflower	1 cup	5.5g
Roasted Potatoes	1 cup	22g	Roasted Radishes	1 cup	4g
Slice of Bread	1 slice	12g	Slice of Keto Bread	1 slice	1g
Bagel	1 plain	54g	FatHead Bagel	1 plain	5g
Waffle	1 waffle	18g	Keto Waffle	1 waffle	5g
Risotto	1 cup	43.5g	Cauliflower Risotto	1 cup	4g

ALL ABOUT THE RECIPES

Are you ready to start cooking? The recipes in this book cover every category of ketogenic cooking. With 200 easy and delicious keto recipes in this book, you will get excited about cooking low-carb, high-fat food and will have plenty of options in each section so that you will never get bored. All the recipes focus on real foods that are easy to find in your favorite grocery store.

I loved coming up with these recipes because, just like you, I want to keep keto easy for my busy lifestyle. You will find that even though these aren't five-ingredient recipes like in my last book, they are still simple and achievable for home cooks of all levels.

Each recipe will be labeled to call out whether it works for those with allergies or sensitivities to certain foods. Look for these labels throughout the recipes to quickly see if a recipe will work for you.

Each recipe also includes a tip, such as how to make a variation on the recipe or how to make it paleo-friendly. Use these tips to help customize your diet to fit your unique situation.

All of the recipes in this book are approved by my daughter, who is my Chief Taste Tester. I love getting her to try new foods, and if she likes something, then I know it is good because she does not hold back! The recipes labeled Comfort Food are some of her absolute favorites because they turn familiar carb-filled favorites into keto-friendly deliciousness.

DAIRY-FREE
(Recipes that do not contain dairy products. Please note that this does not include ghee.)

NUT-FREE
(Recipes that do not contain nuts. Please note that this does not include coconuts.)

ALLERGEN-FREE
(Recipes that do not contain, or can be modified so they don't contain, any of the eight major food allergens: milk, eggs, fish, shellfish, tree nuts, peanuts, wheat, soy.)

PALEO / PALEO-FRIENDLY
(Recipes that are paleo or can be easily altered to be paleo.)

SUPER QUICK
(30 minutes or less, including prep time and cook time.)

COMFORT FOOD
(Common dishes that have been keto-fied or are just generally comforting dishes.)

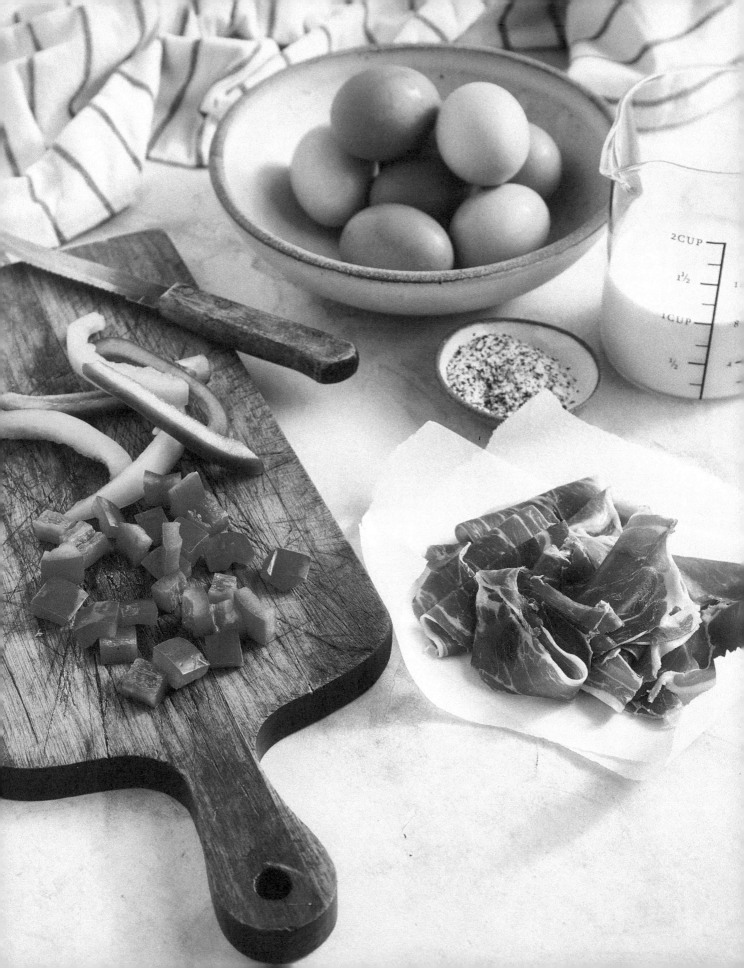

THE MEAL PLANS

CHAPTER TWO

I know it can be confusing to figure out how much fat to incorporate into your diet when you first begin keto. It can be scary to all of a sudden eat a lot of fat, even healthy fat, after being used to a standard American diet. That's why I have provided three two-week meal plans, using recipes from this book, that will offer up suggestions for how to incorporate healthy fats and a diverse assortment of foods into your ketogenic lifestyle. You can follow them closely, or just use them as inspiration. Everyone's body and situation is different, so please feel free to tweak these meal plans to fit your specific needs.

The meal plans are designed to encourage weight loss. They are:

1. Keto Weight Loss Meal Plan **with** Full-Fat Dairy
2. Keto Paleo Weight Loss Meal Plan **without** Full-Fat Dairy
3. Keto Weight Loss Meal Plan **without** the Big 8 Allergens

KETO WEIGHT LOSS MEAL PLAN WITH FULL-FAT DAIRY

This meal plan incorporates healthy fats to keep you full while also allowing you to eat less throughout the day. This meal plan also incorporates intermittent fasting, which means you eat during a six- to eight-hour window and you fast the other 16 to 18 hours. This may sound tough at first, but remember that you are asleep a good chunk of those hours. I follow the Bulletproof Diet's intermittent fasting protocol, which allows a Fatty Latte (page 82), Fatty Iced Coffee (page 84), or Fatty Tea (page 85) in the morning. The high fat content will keep you full and satiated until it's time for lunch, and because it is all fat, your body will be tricked into thinking you are still fasting.

If you are in your first couple weeks of keto, you may find intermittent fasting to be difficult, as your body has not become fat-adapted yet, so you will be hungrier than someone who is three to four weeks into the keto journey. If this sounds like you, feel free to add breakfast food in the morning in addition to a fatty coffee or tea. The meal plans are just to provide some inspiration and guidance, but if your body is telling you it is hungry (or full) please listen and adjust as needed.

The times in the meal plan are based on a "typical work day," but they can be customized for your lifestyle. They are simply meant to demonstrate how to work within your eating window. As mentioned, drinking the fatty coffee or beverage of choice at 8 a.m. should satiate you, especially once you are fat-adapted, but if you need another fatty coffee mid-morning, feel free. If your lunch break is at noon, eat at noon. This example shows 2 p.m. just to get a couple extra hours of fasting in, but any time between noon and 2 p.m. would be great for lunch. In the evening you will stop eating or drinking anything but water by 8 p.m.

- 8 a.m.: Morning drink
- 2 p.m.: Meal 1
- 7 p.m.: Meal 2 + dessert (if applicable)
- Snacks can be anytime you feel hungry before 8 p.m.

Some people on keto do not count calories and others do. As you transition into a ketogenic diet, you might want to consider starting with a slightly higher number of calories than you normally would consume in a day. I know this seems counterintuitive for losing weight, but starting the diet and also restricting calories at the same time may make your transition into ketosis more difficult. Feel free to use the menus as a starting place, and add in an optional snack from the list below the meal plan if you feel hungry. You can always reduce calories once you acclimate to using fat as your new fuel source!

Personally, I like to design my meals to be around 500 to 700 calories. Because I eat two meals a day plus one fatty coffee, it's pretty easy for me to stay within the caloric range that I am comfortable with, which is about 1,500 to 1,800 calories per day, but I have been keto for going on three years. Your activity level also plays a role in this, so check out the many keto macro calculators online to get numbers tailored for your body, goals, and activity level. These meal plans are based on net carbs, not total carbs. As mentioned in chapter 1 (page 2), net carbs is the fiber subtracted from the total carbs. If a recipe includes sweetener, in this case erythritol, the sugar alcohols are not counted. The net carb number is what is actually digested and what has an impact on blood glucose.

If you stick with the same formula as I do, two meals per day plus a fatty coffee, it will be easy for you to make your way through this book and determine which recipes you can pair up to design a daily menu. Feel free to add other sides, snacks, sweets, and beverages to the meal plans if this is not enough food for you. I have listed some no-cook snack options with each meal plan for quick reference. You can also find keto-friendly snacks on your own and incorporate those into these meal plans. Cheese, guacamole packets, and macadamia nuts are some of the convenient snacks I tend to pick up when I'm out and about.

If you ever want to add more fats, you can easily do so by adding MCT oil or drizzling Bulletproof Brain Octane Oil over your food. Both are flavorless and odorless, so they are a great way to easily add quality fats to any meal. Many brands also make convenient to-go single-serving packets that you can keep with you. MCT oil also comes in a powdered variety that can be added to drinks or baked goods. What I hope you take away from these meal plans is that there are a lot of ways to do keto and a huge variety of foods you can eat.

You will see that this menu calls for 3 liters of water per day, and this is super important! There are so many reasons water is beneficial, but one key benefit is that water helps suppress your appetite and curb cravings. Water also helps you metabolize fat faster (and if you are interested in this meal plan, I am guessing you want to burn fat!), so drink up.

KETO PALEO WEIGHT LOSS MEAL PLAN WITHOUT FULL-FAT DAIRY

A keto version of a paleo diet includes whole foods like vegetables, high-quality meat, fish, and poultry. However, it excludes dairy, sweeteners, and carbs that are paleo-friendly but are not keto-paleo-friendly, like sweet potatoes. As with all the meal plans, you can switch out the Fatty Latte with another drink from the snack menu if you wish.

KETO WEIGHT LOSS MEAL PLAN WITHOUT THE BIG 8 ALLERGENS

Food allergies can make any way of eating more complicated, but it is very possible to find success with keto while eliminating the eight major allergens: eggs, wheat, peanuts, tree nuts, milk, fish, shellfish, and soybeans.

This meal plan does include coconut, which is classified as a fruit. The Food and Drug Administration recognizes coconut as a tree nut, but most people allergic to tree nuts can safely eat coconut.

Keto Weight Loss Meal Plan with Full-Fat Dairy • WEEK 1

	MONDAY	TUESDAY	WEDNESDAY
MORNING	Fatty Latte Calories: 423; Total Fat: 47G; Protein: 2G; Total Carbs: 4G; Fiber: 1G; Net Carbs: 3G	Fatty Latte Calories: 423; Total Fat: 47G; Protein: 2G; Total Carbs: 4G; Fiber: 1G; Net Carbs: 3G	Fatty Latte Calories: 423; Total Fat: 47G; Protein: 2G; Total Carbs: 4G; Fiber: 1G; Net Carbs: 3G
MEAL 1	Seaweed Square Pile Ups Calories: 165; Total Fat: 9G; Protein: 19G; Total Carbs: 6G; Fiber: 3G; Net Carbs: 3G	Chopped Buffalo Chicken Salad Calories: 336; Total Fat: 18G; Protein: 27G; Total Carbs: 21G; Fiber: 11G; Net Carbs: 10G	Thai Shrimp and Zoodle Salad Calories: 335; Total Fat: 19G; Protein: 28G; Total Carbs: 13G; Fiber: 4G; Net Carbs: 9G
MEAL 2	Spinach and Artichoke "Dip" Soup Calories: 395; Total Fat: 34G; Protein: 12G; Total Carbs: 14G; Fiber: 2G; Net Carbs: 12G Mexican Cauliflower Rice with Shredded Chicken Calories: 388; Total Fat: 23G; Protein: 28G; Total Carbs: 18G; Fiber: 7G; Net Carbs: 11G	Baked Parmesan Tomatoes Calories: 124; Total Fat: 7G; Protein: 10G; Total Carbs: 5G; Fiber: 1G; Net Carbs: 4G Bacon Cheeseburger Soup Calories: 410; Total Fat: 34G; Protein: 21G; Total Carbs: 5G; Fiber: 1G; Net Carbs: 3G 2 servings Cloud Oopsie Rolls Calories: 410; Total Fat: 34G; Protein: 21G; Total Carbs: 5G; Fiber: 1G; Net Carbs: 3G	Chili-Lime Shrimp Cobb Salad Calories: 741; Total Fat: 53G; Protein: 52G; Total Carbs: 14G; Fiber: 8G; Net Carbs: 6G
DESSERT	Keto Cream Cheese "Fluff" Calories: 219; Total Fat: 22G; Protein: 3G; Total Carbs: 1G; Fiber: 0G; Net Carbs: 1G	Berry-Coconut Chia Pudding Calories: 288; Total Fat: 24G; Protein: 4G; Total Carbs: 11G; Fiber: 6G; Net Carbs: 5G	Pecan Fat Bomb Calories: 181; Total Fat: 19G; Protein: 1G; Total Carbs: 3G; Fiber: 2G; Net Carbs: 1G
DRINK	3L water	3L water	3L water
TOTAL	Fat (135G)..............76.4% Protein (64G)...........16.1% Carbs (30G net)..........7.5% Calories: 1590	Fat (134G)..............74.3% Protein (66G)...........16.2% Carbs (25G net)..........9.5% Calories: 1623	Fat (138G)..............73.9% Protein (83G)...........19.8% Carbs (19G net)..........6.3% Calories: 1680

+ Additional snack if desired

THURSDAY	FRIDAY	SATURDAY	SUNDAY
Fatty Latte Calories: 423; Total Fat: 47G; Protein: 2G; Total Carbs: 4G; Fiber: 1G; Net Carbs: 3G	**Fatty Latte** Calories: 423; Total Fat: 47G; Protein: 2G; Total Carbs: 4G; Fiber: 1G; Net Carbs: 3G	**Fatty Latte** Calories: 423; Total Fat: 47G; Protein: 2G; Total Carbs: 4G; Fiber: 1G; Net Carbs: 3G	**Fatty Latte** Calories: 423; Total Fat: 47G; Protein: 2G; Total Carbs: 4G; Fiber: 1G; Net Carbs: 3G
Slow Cooker Chicken Enchilada Bowls Calories: 427; Total Fat: 28G; Protein: 30G; Total Carbs: 13G; Fiber: 7G; Net Carbs: 6G	**Mediterranean Burger** Calories: 531; Total Fat: 42G; Protein: 33G; Total Carbs: 7G; Fiber: 3G; Net Carbs: 4G	**2 FatHead Sausage Breakfast Biscuits** Calories: 229; Total Fat: 18G; Protein: 16G; Total Carbs: 1G; Fiber: 0G; Net Carbs: 1G	**Bacon-Wrapped Cheese "Fries"** Calories: 184; Total Fat: 14G; Protein: 12G; Total Carbs: 1G; Fiber: 0G; Net Carbs: 1G **Cheesy Spinach Egg Bake with Pork Rind Dust** Calories: 338; Total Fat: 26G; Protein: 25G; Total Carbs: 3G; Fiber: 1G; Net Carbs: 2G
BAE (Bacon, Avocado, Egg) Butter Lettuce Salad Calories: 313; Total Fat: 26G; Protein: 15G; Total Carbs: 9G; Fiber: 6G; Net Carbs: 3G **Bacon-Wrapped Pickle "Fries"** Calories: 190; Total Fat: 14G; Protein: 13G; Total Carbs: 4G; Fiber: 2G; Net Carbs: 2G	**Prosciutto-Wrapped Cod** Calories: 317; Total Fat: 18G; Protein: 38G; Total Carbs: 0G; Fiber: 0G; Net Carbs: 0G **2 servings Creamy Cucumber Salad** Calories: 118; Total Fat: 6G; Protein: 3G; Total Carbs: 13G; Fiber: 2G; Net Carbs: 11G	**Salmon Burgers with Chive Aioli and Greens** Calories: 471; Total Fat: 31G; Protein: 38G; Total Carbs: 10G; Fiber: 2G; Net Carbs: 8G	**Dairy-Free Chicken Alfredo with Mushrooms** Calories: 464; Total Fat: 36G; Protein: 22G; Total Carbs: 13G; Fiber: 3G; Net Carbs: 10G
Blueberry-Lemon Cake Calories: 147; Total Fat: 11G; Protein: 5G; Total Carbs: 5G; Fiber: 3G; Net Carbs: 2G **Pink Passion Iced Tea** Calories: 114; Total Fat: 12G; Protein: 1G; Total Carbs: 2G; Fiber: 0G; Net Carbs: 2G	**2 Spicy Chocolate Fat Bombs** Calories: 190; Total Fat: 18G; Protein: 2G; Total Carbs: 5G; Fiber: 3G; Net Carbs: 2G	**Nut Butter Chocolate Chip Cookies** Calories: 245; Total Fat: 17G; Protein: 5G; Total Carbs: 8G; Fiber: 3G; Net Carbs: 5G **Pink Passion Iced Tea** Calories: 114; Total Fat: 12G; Protein: 1G; Total Carbs: 2G; Fiber: 0G; Net Carbs: 2G	**Nut Butter Chocolate Chip Cookies** Calories: 245; Total Fat: 17G; Protein: 5G; Total Carbs: 8G; Fiber: 3G; Net Carbs: 5G
3L water	3L water	3L water	3L water
Fat (138G) .... 76.9%, Protein (66G) .... 16.4% Carbs (18G net) .... 6.7% Calories: 1614	Fat (131G) .... 74.7% Protein (68G) .... 17.2% Carbs (20G net) .... 8.1% Calories: 1579	Fat (125G) .... 75.9% Protein (62G) .... 16.7% Carbs (19G net) .... 7.4% Calories: 1482	Fat (140G) .... 76.2% Protein (66G) .... 16% Carbs (21G net) .... 7.8% Calories: 1654

Keto Weight Loss Meal Plan with Full-Fat Dairy • WEEK 2

	MONDAY	TUESDAY	WEDNESDAY
MORNING	Fatty Latte Calories: 423; Total Fat: 47G; Protein: 2G; Total Carbs: 4G; Fiber: 1G; Net Carbs: 3G	Fatty Latte Calories: 423; Total Fat: 47G; Protein: 2G; Total Carbs: 4G; Fiber: 1G; Net Carbs: 3G	Fatty Latte Calories: 423; Total Fat: 47G; Protein: 2G; Total Carbs: 4G; Fiber: 1G; Net Carbs: 3G
MEAL 1	Spinach and Artichoke "Dip" Soup Calories: 427; Total Fat: 28G; Protein: 30G; Total Carbs: 13G; Fiber: 7G; Net Carbs: 6G Antipasto Salad Calories: 240; Total Fat: 18G; Protein: 9G; Total Carbs: 14G; Fiber: 8G; Net Carbs: 6G	Chopped Buffalo Chicken Salad Calories: 336; Total Fat: 18G; Protein: 27G; Total Carbs: 21G; Fiber: 11G; Net Carbs: 10G	Avocado Cotija Salad Calories: 454; Total Fat: 39G; Protein: 8G; Total Carbs: 27G; Fiber: 12G; Net Carbs: 15G
MEAL 2	Slow Cooker Chili With Bacon Calories: 399; Total Fat: 27G; Protein: 30G; Total Carbs: 9G; Fiber: 1G; Net Carbs: 8G	Herb and Dijon Pork Chops Calories: 323; Total Fat: 22G; Protein: 27G; Total Carbs: 3G; Fiber: 0G; Net Carbs: 3G Kale and Butternut Squash Gratin Calories: 266; Total Fat: 22G; Protein: 8G; Total Carbs: 9G; Fiber: 2G; Net Carbs: 7G	Oven-Baked Garlic and Herb Steak Calories: 609; Total Fat: 48G; Protein: 36G; Total Carbs: 6G; Fiber: 2G; Net Carbs: 4G
DESSERT		Keto Cream Cheese "Fluff" Calories: 219; Total Fat: 22G; Protein: 3G; Total Carbs: 1G; Fiber: 0G; Net Carbs: 1G	Chocolate Cookie Bark Calories: 130; Total Fat: 10G; Protein: 4G; Total Carbs: 6G; Fiber: 3G; Net Carbs: 3G
DRINK	3L water	3L water	3L water
TOTAL	Fat (126G)............... 77.8% Protein (53G)............ 14.6% Carbs (29G net)........... 7.6% Calories: 1457	Fat (131G)............... 75.2% Protein (67G)............. 17.1% Carbs (24G net)............7.7% Calories: 1567	Fat (144G)............... 80.2% Protein (50G)............ 12.4% Carbs (25G net)........... 7.4% Calories: 1616

+ Additional snack if desired

Examples of no-cook snacks:

Pepperoni "Tacos"
Calories: 262; Total Fat: 23G;
Protein: 10G; Total Carbs: 3G;
Fiber: 1G; Net Carbs: 2G

Seaweed Square Pile Ups
Calories: 165; Total Fat: 9G;
Protein: 19G; Total Carbs: 6G;
Fiber: 3G; Net Carbs: 3G

Salmon Avocado Boats
Calories: 188; Total Fat: 14G;
Protein: 7G; Total Carbs: 11G;
Fiber: 5G; Net Carbs: 6G

Berry-Coconut Chia Pudding
Calories: 288; Total Fat: 24G;
Protein: 4G; Total Carbs: 11G;
Fiber: 6G; Net Carbs: 5G

Pecan Fat Bomb
Calories: 181; Total Fat: 19G;
Protein: 1G; Total Carbs: 3G;
Fiber: 2G; Net Carbs: 1G

THURSDAY	FRIDAY	SATURDAY	SUNDAY
Fatty Latte Calories: 423; Total Fat: 47G; Protein: 2G; Total Carbs: 4G; Fiber: 1G; Net Carbs: 3G	**Fatty Latte** Calories: 423; Total Fat: 47G; Protein: 2G; Total Carbs: 4G; Fiber: 1G; Net Carbs: 3G	**Fatty Latte** Calories: 423; Total Fat: 47G; Protein: 2G; Total Carbs: 4G; Fiber: 1G; Net Carbs: 3G	**Fatty Latte** Calories: 423; Total Fat: 47G; Protein: 2G; Total Carbs: 4G; Fiber: 1G; Net Carbs: 3G
Portobello Breakfast Cups Calories: 308; Total Fat: 21G; Protein: 23G; Total Carbs: 10G; Fiber: 2G; Net Carbs: 8G **Buffalo "Wing" Deviled Eggs** Calories: 223; Total Fat: 19G Protein: 11G; Total Carbs: 2G; Fiber: 1G; Net Carbs: 1G	**Mediterranean Wedge Salad** Calories: 196; Total Fat: 17G; Protein: 2G; Total Carbs: 12G; Fiber: 3G; Net Carbs: 9G **Mozzarella Prosciutto Bombs** Calories: 450; Total Fat: 35G; Protein: 31G; Total Carbs: 2G; Fiber: 1G; Net Carbs: 1G	**Sheet Pan Steak and Eggs** Calories: 409; Total Fat: 29G; Protein: 33G; Total Carbs: 4G; Fiber: 2G; Net Carbs: 2G	**Bacon-Wrapped Pork Nuggets** Calories: 353; Total Fat: 30G; Protein: 20G; Total Carbs: 1G; Fiber: 0G; Net Carbs: 1G **Prosciutto-Wrapped Peppers** Calories: 236; Total Fat: 16G; Protein: 12G; Total Carbs: 11G; Fiber: 2G; Net Carbs: 9G
Pork Butter Burger Calories: 504; Total Fat: 44G; Protein: 27G; Total Carbs: 0G; Fiber: 0G; Net Carbs: 0G **Cloud Oopsie Rolls** Calories: 42; Total Fat: 4G; Protein: 2G; Total Carbs: 0G; Fiber: 0G; Net Carbs: 0G	**Sheet Pan Fajitas** Calories: 426; Total Fat: 30G; Protein: 26G; Total Carbs: 13G; Fiber: 3G; Net Carbs: 10G	**Pepperoni and Pepperoncini FatHead Pizza** Calories: 416; Total Fat: 33G; Protein: 25G; Total Carbs: 5G; Fiber: 1G; Net Carbs: 4G	**Green Chile Meatballs** Calories: 326; Total Fat: 22G; Protein: 26G; Total Carbs: 6G; Fiber: 1G; Net Carbs: 5G **Roasted Veggies** Calories: 83; Total Fat: 7G; Protein: 2G; Total Carbs: 5G; Fiber: 2G; Net Carbs: 3G
	Blueberry-Lemon Cake Calories: 147; Total Fat: 11G; Protein: 5G; Total Carbs: 5G; Fiber: 3G; Net Carbs: 2G	**Blueberry-Lemon Cake** Calories: 147; Total Fat: 11G; Protein: 5G; Total Carbs: 5G; Fiber: 3G; Net Carbs: 2G **Pink Passion Iced Tea** Calories: 114; Total Fat: 12G; Protein: 1G; Total Carbs: 2G; Fiber: 0G; Net Carbs: 2G	**Blueberry-Lemon Cake** Calories: 147; Total Fat: 11G; Protein: 5G; Total Carbs: 5G; Fiber: 3G; Net Carbs: 2G
3L water	3L water	3L water	3L water
Fat (118G) .... 70.8% **Protein (65G)** .... 17.3% **Carbs (12G net)** .... 11.9% Calories: 1500	**Fat (140G)** .... 76.7% **Protein (66G)** .... 16.1% **Carbs (25G net)** .... 7.2% Calories: 1642	**Fat (132G)** .... 78.7% **Protein (66G)** .... 17.5% **Carbs (13G net)** .... 3.8% Calories: 1509	**Fat (133G)** .... 76.3% **Protein (67G)** .... 17.1% **Carbs (23G net)** .... 6.6% Calories: 1568

Spicy Chocolate Fat Bomb
Calories: 190; Total Fat: 18G;
Protein: 2G; Total Carbs: 5G;
Fiber: 3G; Net Carbs: 2G

Pink Passion Iced Tea
Calories: 114; Total Fat: 12G;
Protein: 1G; Total Carbs: 2G;
Fiber: 0G; Net Carbs: 2G

Nut Butter Smoothie
Calories: 330; Total Fat: 34G;
Protein: 5G; Total Carbs: 7G;
Fiber: 1G; Net Carbs: 6G

Avocado Turmeric Smoothie
Calories: 239; Total Fat: 23G;
Protein: 3G; Total Carbs: 9G;
Fiber: 5G; Net Carbs: 4G

Keto Cream Cheese "Fluff"
Calories: 219; Total Fat: 22G;
Protein: 3G; Total Carbs: 1G;
Fiber: 0G; Net Carbs: 1G

Keto Paleo Weight Loss Meal Plan without Full-Fat Dairy • WEEK 1

	MONDAY	TUESDAY	WEDNESDAY
MORNING	**Fatty Latte** Calories: 423; Total Fat: 47G; Protein: 2G; Total Carbs: 4G; Fiber: 1G; Net Carbs: 3G	**Fatty Latte** Calories: 423; Total Fat: 47G; Protein: 2G; Total Carbs: 4G; Fiber: 1G; Net Carbs: 3G	**Fatty Latte** Calories: 423; Total Fat: 47G; Protein: 2G; Total Carbs: 4G; Fiber: 1G; Net Carbs: 3G
MEAL 1	**Spicy Shrimp with Shirataki Noodles** Calories: 240; Total Fat: 15G; Protein: 19G; Total Carbs: 8G; Fiber: 2G; Net Carbs: 6G	**Ground Pork Egg Roll Slaw** Calories: 423; Total Fat: 33G; Protein: 22G; Total Carbs: 10G; Fiber: 3G; Net Carbs: 7G	**Spicy Slow Cooker Shredded Pork** Calories: 412; Total Fat: 26G; Protein: 40G; Total Carbs: 6G; Fiber: 2G; Net Carbs: 4G
MEAL 2	**Garlic, Mushroom, and Bacon Burger** Calories: 382; Total Fat: 28G; Protein: 30G; Total Carbs: 4G; Fiber: 1G; Net Carbs: 3G **Antipasto Salad** Calories: 240; Total Fat: 18G; Protein: 9G; Total Carbs: 14G; Fiber: 8G; Net Carbs: 6G	**Sheet Pan Steak and Eggs** Calories: 409; Total Fat: 29G; Protein: 33G; Total Carbs: 4G; Fiber: 2G; Net Carbs: 2G	**Vietnamese Steak Cauliflower and Rice Bowl** Calories: 466; Total Fat: 34G; Protein: 34G; Total Carbs: 6G; Fiber: 1G; Net Carbs: 5G
DESSERT	**Keto-Chata** Calories: 131; Total Fat: 13G; Protein: 1G; Total Carbs: 5G; Fiber: 1G; Net Carbs: 4G	**Nut Butter Smoothie** Calories: 330; Total Fat: 34G; Protein: 5G; Total Carbs: 7G; Fiber: 1G; Net Carbs: 6G	**Fatty Hot Chocolate** Calories: 465; Total Fat: 49G; Protein: 6G; Total Carbs: 14G; Fiber: 3G; Net Carbs: 11G
DRINK	3L water	3L water	3L water
TOTAL	Fat (121G) .... 76.9% Protein (61G) .... 17.2% Carbs (22G net) .... 5.9% Calories: 1416	Fat (143G) .... 79.2% Protein (62G) .... 15.6% Carbs (18G net) .... 5.2% Calories: 1585	Fat (156G) .... 80.5% Protein (82G) .... 16.6% Carbs (23G net) .... 2.9% Calories: 1766

+ Additional snack if desired

Examples of keto paleo
no-cook snacks:

Fatty Latte
Calories: 423; Total Fat: 47G;
Protein: 2G; Total Carbs: 4G;
Fiber: 1G; Net Carbs: 3G

Fatty Iced Coffee
Calories: 189; Total Fat: 21G;
Protein: 1G; Total Carbs: 2G;
Fiber: 0G; Net Carbs: 2G

Fatty Hot Chocolate
Calories: 465; Total Fat: 49G;
Protein: 6G; Total Carbs: 14G;
Fiber: 3G; Net Carbs: 11G

Fatty Pumpkin Spice Latte
Calories: 409; Total Fat: 45G;
Protein: 3G; Total Carbs: 6G;
Fiber: 1G; Net Carbs: 5G

Fatty Tea
Calories: 155; Total Fat: 12G;
Protein: 11G; Total Carbs: 1G;
Fiber: 1G; Net Carbs: 0G

Fatty Matcha
Calories: 163; Total Fat: 17G;
Protein: 2G; Total Carbs: 3G;
Fiber: 1G; Net Carbs: 2G

THURSDAY	FRIDAY	SATURDAY	SUNDAY
Fatty Latte Calories: 423; Total Fat: 47G; Protein: 2G; Total Carbs: 4G; Fiber: 1G; Net Carbs: 3G	**Fatty Latte** Calories: 423; Total Fat: 47G; Protein: 2G; Total Carbs: 4G; Fiber: 1G; Net Carbs: 3G	**Fatty Latte** Calories: 423; Total Fat: 47G; Protein: 2G; Total Carbs: 4G; Fiber: 1G; Net Carbs: 3G	**Fatty Latte** Calories: 423; Total Fat: 47G; Protein: 2G; Total Carbs: 4G; Fiber: 1G; Net Carbs: 3G
Spicy Tuna Poke Bowl Calories: 518; Total Fat: 34G; Protein: 37G; Total Carbs: 16G; Fiber: 10G; Net Carbs: 6G	**Crunchy Thai Chicken Salad** Calories: 354; Total Fat: 18G; Protein: 38G; Total Carbs: 12G; Fiber: 4G; Net Carbs: 8G	**Baked Chorizo Eggs** Calories: 321; Total Fat: 24G; Protein: 19G; Total Carbs: 10G; Fiber: 2G; Net Carbs: 8G **Bacon-Wrapped Avocado "Fries"** Calories: 286; Total Fat: 24G; Protein: 13G; Total Carbs: 6G; Fiber: 5G; Net Carbs: 1G	**Smoked Salmon Eggs Benedict** Calories: 323; Total Fat: 23G; Protein: 29G; Total Carbs: 0G; Fiber: 0G; Net Carbs: 0G
Sheet Pan Fajitas Calories: 426; Total Fat: 30G; Protein: 26G; Total Carbs: 13G; Fiber: 3G; Net Carbs: 10G **Dairy-Free Avocado Crema** Calories: 206; Total Fat: 20G; Protein: 2G; Total Carbs: 7G; Fiber: 5G; Net Carbs: 2G	**Bacon-Wrapped Pork Nuggets** Calories: 353; Total Fat: 30G; Protein: 20G; Total Carbs: 1G; Fiber: 0G; Net Carbs: 1G **Cucumber Bites** Calories: 95; Total Fat: 7G; Protein: 3G; Total Carbs: 6G; Fiber: 1G; Net Carbs: 5G	**Sriracha Pork Stir-Fry** Calories: 469; Total Fat: 38G; Protein: 24G; Total Carbs: 11G; Fiber: 4G; Net Carbs: 7G	**Fajita-Spiced Skirt Steak with Mexican Cauliflower Rice** Calories: 355; Total Fat: 23G; Protein: 26G; Total Carbs: 11G; Fiber: 4G; Net Carbs: 7G
	Mint Cacao Chip Smoothie Calories: 415; Total Fat: 41G; Protein: 5G; Total Carbs: 16G; Fiber: 7G; Net Carbs: 9G	**Keto-Chata** Calories: 131; Total Fat: 13G; Protein: 1G; Total Carbs: 5G; Fiber: 1G; Net Carbs: 4G	**Blueberry-Coconut Smoothie** Calories: 506; Total Fat: 53G; Protein: 5G; Total Carbs: 12G; Fiber: 1G; Net Carbs: 11G
3L water	3L water	3L water	3L water
Fat (131G) . . . . 74.9% **Protein (67G)** . . . . 17% **Carbs (21G net)** . . . . 8.1% Calories: 1573	**Fat (143G)** . . . . 78.5% **Protein (68G)** . . . . 16.6% **Carbs (26G net)** . . . . 4.9% Calories: 1640	**Fat (146G)** . . . . 80% **Protein (59G)** . . . . 14.5% **Carbs (23G net)** . . . . 5.5% Calories: 1630	**Fat (146G)** . . . . 80.1% **Protein (63G)** . . . . 14.6% **Carbs (21G net)** . . . . 5.3% Calories: 1607

Pink Passion Iced Tea
Calories: 114; Total Fat: 12G;
Protein: 1G; Total Carbs: 2G;
Fiber: 0G; Net Carbs: 2G

Blueberry-Coconut Smoothie
Calories: 506; Total Fat: 53G;
Protein: 5G; Total Carbs: 12G;
Fiber: 1G; Net Carbs: 11G

Cacao Crunch Cereal
Per Serving (Cereal Only):
Calories: 325; Total Fat: 27G;
Protein: 10G; Total Carbs: 17G;
Fiber: 12G; Net Carbs: 5G

Nut Butter Smoothie
Calories: 330; Total Fat: 34G;
Protein: 5G; Total Carbs: 7G;
Fiber: 1G; Net Carbs: 6G

Mint Cacao Chip Smoothie
Calories: 415; Total Fat: 41G;
Protein: 5G; Total Carbs: 16G;
Fiber: 7G; Net Carbs: 9G

Keto-Chata
Calories: 131; Total Fat: 13G;
Protein: 1G; Total Carbs: 5G;
Fiber: 1G; Net Carbs: 4G

Keto Paleo Weight Loss Meal Plan without Full-Fat Dairy • WEEK 2

	MONDAY	TUESDAY	WEDNESDAY
MORNING	**Fatty Latte** Calories: 423; Total Fat: 47G; Protein: 2G; Total Carbs: 4G; Fiber: 1G; Net Carbs: 3G	**Fatty Latte** Calories: 423; Total Fat: 47G; Protein: 2G; Total Carbs: 4G; Fiber: 1G; Net Carbs: 3G	**Fatty Latte** Calories: 423; Total Fat: 47G; Protein: 2G; Total Carbs: 4G; Fiber: 1G; Net Carbs: 3G
MEAL 1	**Creamy Green Chile Chicken Soup** Calories: 325; Total Fat: 21G; Protein: 25G; Total Carbs: 9G; Fiber: 2G; Net Carbs: 7G	**Bacon-Strawberry Spinach Salad** Calories: 380; Total Fat: 34G; Protein: 12G; Total Carbs: 10G; Fiber: 6G; Net Carbs: 4G	**Green Chile Meatballs** Calories: 326; Total Fat: 22G; Protein: 26G; Total Carbs: 6G; Fiber: 1G; Net Carbs: 5G **Mediterranean Wedge Salad** Calories: 196; Total Fat: 17G; Protein: 2G; Total Carbs: 12G; Fiber: 3G; Net Carbs: 9G
MEAL 2	**Salmon Burgers with Chive Aioli and Greens** Calories: 471; Total Fat: 31G; Protein: 38G; Total Carbs: 10G; Fiber: 2G; Net Carbs: 8G **Roasted Veggies** Calories: 83; Total Fat: 7G; Protein: 2G; Total Carbs: 5G; Fiber: 2G; Net Carbs: 3G	**Prosciutto-Wrapped Cod** Calories: 317; Total Fat: 18G; Protein: 38G; Total Carbs: 0G; Fiber: 0G; Net Carbs: 0G **2 Crab-Stuffed Mushrooms** Calories: 139; Total Fat: 10G; Protein: 8G; Total Carbs: 3G; Fiber: 1G; Net Carbs: 2G	**"Spaghetti" and Meat Sauce** Calories: 495; Total Fat: 39G; Protein: 24G; Total Carbs: 11G; Fiber: 3G; Net Carbs: 8G
DESSERT	**Fatty Latte** Calories: 423; Total Fat: 47G; Protein: 2G; Total Carbs: 4G; Fiber: 1G; Net Carbs: 3G	**Keto-Chata** Calories: 131; Total Fat: 13G; Protein: 1G; Total Carbs: 5G; Fiber: 1G; Net Carbs: 4G	
DRINK	3L water	3L water	3L water
TOTAL	Fat (153G)................ 78.8% Protein (69G)............. 16% Carbs (24G net) .... 5.2% Calories: 1725	Fat (122G)................ 77.9% Protein (61G)............. 17.5% Carbs (13G net) .... 4.6% Calories: 1390	Fat (125G) .... 78.1% Protein (54G)............. 15% Carbs (25G net).......... 6.9% Calories: 1440

+ Additional snack if desired

THURSDAY	FRIDAY	SATURDAY	SUNDAY
Fatty Latte Calories: 423; Total Fat: 47G; Protein: 2G; Total Carbs: 4G; Fiber: 1G; Net Carbs: 3G	**Fatty Latte** Calories: 423; Total Fat: 47G; Protein: 2G; Total Carbs: 4G; Fiber: 1G; Net Carbs: 3G	**Fatty Latte** Calories: 423; Total Fat: 47G; Protein: 2G; Total Carbs: 4G; Fiber: 1G; Net Carbs: 3G	**Fatty Latte** Calories: 423; Total Fat: 47G; Protein: 2G; Total Carbs: 4G; Fiber: 1G; Net Carbs: 3G
Thai Shrimp and Zoodle Salad Calories: 335; Total Fat: 19G; Protein: 28G; Total Carbs: 13G; Fiber: 4G; Net Carbs: 9G	**Pork Burger Lettuce Cups** Calories: 395; Total Fat: 33G; Protein: 20G; Total Carbs: 5G; Fiber: 1G; Net Carbs: 4G	**Salmon Avocado Boats** Calories: 188; Total Fat: 14G; Protein: 7G; Total Carbs: 11G; Fiber: 5G; Net Carbs: 6G	**Bacon and Egg Breakfast Jars** Calories: 507; Total Fat: 43G; Protein: 26G; Total Carbs: 5G; Fiber: 1G; Net Carbs: 4G
Bacon-Wrapped Steak Bites with Mustard Dipping Sauce Calories: 419; Total Fat: 31G; Protein: 30G; Total Carbs: 4G; Fiber: 0G; Net Carbs: 4G	**2 Broiled Lobster Tails** Calories: 285; Total Fat: 24G; Protein: 17G; Total Carbs: 2G; Fiber: 1G; Net Carbs: 1G **Lemony Spinach** Calories: 82; Total Fat: 7G; Protein: 2G; Total Carbs: 4G; Fiber: 2G; Net Carbs: 2G	**Bacon-Wrapped Pork Loin** Calories: 447; Total Fat: 34G; Protein: 33G; Total Carbs: 0G; Fiber: 0G; Net Carbs: 0G	**Slow Cooker Steak and Mushroom Bites** Calories: 594; Total Fat: 52G; Protein: 29G; Total Carbs: 5G; Fiber: 1G; Net Carbs: 4G **Roasted Veggies** Calories: 83; Total Fat: 7G; Protein: 2G; Total Carbs: 5G; Fiber: 2G; Net Carbs: 3G
Mint Cacao Chip Smoothie Calories: 415; Total Fat: 41G; Protein: 5G; Total Carbs: 16G; Fiber: 7G; Net Carbs: 9G		**Cacao Crunch Cereal** Per Serving (Cereal Only): Calories: 325; Total Fat: 27G; Protein: 10G; Total Carbs: 17G; Fiber: 12G; Net Carbs: 5G **Pink Passion Iced Tea** Calories: 114; Total Fat: 12G; Protein: 1G; Total Carbs: 2G; Fiber: 0G; Net Carbs: 2G	
3L water	3L water	3L water	3L water
Fat (138G) .... 78% Protein (65G) .... 16.3% Carbs (25G net) .... 5.7% Calories: 1592	Fat (111G)............. 83.3% Protein (41G)........... 12.8% Carbs (10G net) .... 3.9% Calories: 1185	Fat (134G) .... 79.5% Protein (53G) .... 14.1% Carbs (16G net) .... 6.4% Calories: 1497	Fat (149G) .... 80.2% Protein (59G) .... 14.1% Carbs (14G net) .... 5.7% Calories: 1670

Keto Weight Loss Meal Plan without the Big 8 Allergens • WEEK 1

	MONDAY	TUESDAY	WEDNESDAY
MORNING	Fatty Latte Calories: 423; Total Fat: 47G; Protein: 2G; Total Carbs: 4G; Fiber: 1G; Net Carbs: 3G	Fatty Latte Calories: 423; Total Fat: 47G; Protein: 2G; Total Carbs: 4G; Fiber: 1G; Net Carbs: 3G	Fatty Latte Calories: 423; Total Fat: 47G; Protein: 2G; Total Carbs: 4G; Fiber: 1G; Net Carbs: 3G
MEAL 1	Italian Wraps Calories: 402; Total Fat: 30G; Protein: 27G; Total Carbs: 6G; Fiber: 2G; Net Carbs: 4G	Salmon Avocado Boats Calories: 188; Total Fat: 14G; Protein: 7G; Total Carbs: 11G; Fiber: 5G; Net Carbs: 6G	Avocado Chicken Salad Calories: 308; Total Fat: 17G; Protein: 29G; Total Carbs: 10G; Fiber: 5G; Net Carbs: 5G **Cucumber Bites** Calories: 95; Total Fat: 7G; Protein: 3G; Total Carbs: 6G; Fiber: 1G; Net Carbs: 5G
MEAL 2	Spicy Slow Cooker Shredded Pork (on top of nachos) Calories: 412; Total Fat: 26G; Protein: 40G; Total Carbs: 6G; Fiber: 2G; Net Carbs: 4G **Cheeseless Roasted Cauliflower Nachos** Calories: 288; Total Fat: 24G; Protein: 4G; Total Carbs: 14G; Fiber: 7G; Net Carbs: 7G	"Spaghetti" and Meat Sauce Calories: 495; Total Fat: 39G; Protein: 24G; Total Carbs: 11G; Fiber: 3G; Net Carbs: 8G	Garlic, Mushroom, and Bacon Burger Calories: 382; Total Fat: 28G; Protein: 30G; Total Carbs: 4G; Fiber: 1G; Net Carbs: 3G **Bacon-Wrapped Avocado "Fries"** Calories: 286; Total Fat: 24G; Protein: 13G; Total Carbs: 6G; Fiber: 5G; Net Carbs: 1G
DESSERT		Blueberry-Coconut Smoothie Calories: 506; Total Fat: 53G; Protein: 5G; Total Carbs: 12G; Fiber: 1G; Net Carbs: 11G	
DRINK	3L water	3L water	3L water
TOTAL	Fat (127G) .... 75% Protein (73G) .... 19.1% Carbs (18G net) .... 5.9% Calories: 1525	Fat (153G) .... 85.4% Protein (38G) .... 9.4% Carbs (28G net) .... 5.2% Calories: 1612	Fat (123G) .... 74.1% Protein (77G) .... 20.6% Carbs (17G net) .... 5.3% Calories: 1494

+ Additional snack if desired

Examples of no-cook snacks without the big 8 allergens:

Fatty Latte
Calories: 423; Total Fat: 47G;
Protein: 2G; Total Carbs: 4G;
Fiber: 1G; Net Carbs: 3G

Fatty Iced Coffee
Calories: 189; Total Fat: 21G;
Protein: 1G; Total Carbs: 2G;
Fiber: 0G; Net Carbs: 2G

Fatty Hot Chocolate
Calories: 465; Total Fat: 49G;
Protein: 6G; Total Carbs: 14G;
Fiber: 3G; Net Carbs: 11G

Fatty Pumpkin Spice Latte
Calories: 409; Total Fat: 45G;
Protein: 3G; Total Carbs: 6G;
Fiber: 1G; Net Carbs: 5G

Fatty Tea
Calories: 155; Total Fat: 12G;
Protein: 11G; Total Carbs: 1G;
Fiber: 1G; Net Carbs: 0G

THURSDAY	FRIDAY	SATURDAY	SUNDAY
Fatty Latte Calories: 423; Total Fat: 47G; Protein: 2G; Total Carbs: 4G; Fiber: 1G; Net Carbs: 3G	**Fatty Latte** Calories: 423; Total Fat: 47G; Protein: 2G; Total Carbs: 4G; Fiber: 1G; Net Carbs: 3G	**Fatty Latte** Calories: 423; Total Fat: 47G; Protein: 2G; Total Carbs: 4G; Fiber: 1G; Net Carbs: 3G	**Fatty Latte** Calories: 423; Total Fat: 47G; Protein: 2G; Total Carbs: 4G; Fiber: 1G; Net Carbs: 3G
Ground Pork Egg Roll Slaw Calories: 423; Total Fat: 33G; Protein: 22G; Total Carbs: 10G; Fiber: 3G; Net Carbs: 7G	**Bacon-Strawberry Spinach Salad** Calories: 380; Total Fat: 34G; Protein: 12G; Total Carbs: 10G; Fiber: 6G; Net Carbs: 4G	**Slow Cooker Cauliflower "Fried" Rice** Calories: 184; Total Fat: 12G; Protein: 10G; Total Carbs: 9G; Fiber: 3G; Net Carbs: 6G **Bacon-Wrapped Pickle "Fries"** Calories: 190; Total Fat: 14G; Protein: 13G; Total Carbs: 4G; Fiber: 2G; Net Carbs: 2G	**Asian Beef "Noodle" Bowls** Calories: 404; Total Fat: 31G; Protein: 25G; Total Carbs: 9G; Fiber: 2G; Net Carbs: 7G
Dairy-Free Chicken Alfredo with Mushrooms Calories: 464; Total Fat: 36G; Protein: 22G; Total Carbs: 13G; Fiber: 3G; Net Carbs: 10G **Roasted Cauliflower with Bacon** Calories: 352; Total Fat: 32G; Protein: 9G; Total Carbs: 8G; Fiber: 4G; Net Carbs: 4G	**Slow Cooker Steak and Mushroom Bites** Calories: 594; Total Fat: 52G; Protein: 29G; Total Carbs: 5G; Fiber: 1G; Net Carbs: 4G **Lemony Spinach** Calories: 82; Total Fat: 7G; Protein: 2G; Total Carbs: 4G; Fiber: 2G; Net Carbs: 2G	**Slow Cooker Buffalo Wings** Calories: 603; Total Fat: 48G; Protein: 42G; Total Carbs: 0G; Fiber: 0G; Net Carbs: 0G	**Bacon-Wrapped Steak Bites with Mustard Dipping Sauce** Calories: 419; Total Fat: 31G; Protein: 30G; Total Carbs: 4G; Fiber: 0G; Net Carbs: 4G
	Pink Passion Iced Tea Calories: 114; Total Fat: 12G; Protein: 1G; Total Carbs: 2G; Fiber: 0G; Net Carbs: 2G	**Fatty Hot Chocolate** Calories: 465; Total Fat: 49G; Protein: 6G; Total Carbs: 14G; Fiber: 3G; Net Carbs: 11G	**Pink Passion Iced Tea** Calories: 114; Total Fat: 12G; Protein: 1G; Total Carbs: 2G; Fiber: 0G; Net Carbs: 2G
3L water	3L water	3L water	3L water
Fat (148G) .... 80.1% **Protein (55G)** .... 13.2% **Carbs (24G net)** .... 6.7% Calories: 1662	**Fat (152G)** .... 83.8% **Protein (46G)** .... 11.5% **Carbs (15G net)** .... 5% Calories: 1593	**Fat (170G)** .... 80.1% **Protein (73G)** .... 15.7% **Carbs (22G net)** .... 4.2% Calories: 1865	**Fat (121G)** .... 79.1% **Protein (58G)** .... 17.1% **Carbs (16G net)** .... 3.8% Calories: 1360

Fatty Matcha
Calories: 163; Total Fat: 17G;
Protein: 2G; Total Carbs: 3G;
Fiber: 1G; Net Carbs: 2G

Pink Passion Iced Tea
Calories: 114; Total Fat: 12G;
Protein: 1G; Total Carbs: 2G;
Fiber: 0G; Net Carbs: 2G

Berry Coconut Chia Pudding
Calories: 288; Total Fat: 24G;
Protein: 4G; Total Carbs: 14G;
Fiber: 6G; Net Carbs: 8G

Blueberry-Coconut Smoothie
Calories: 506; Total Fat: 53G;
Protein: 5G; Total Carbs: 12G;
Fiber: 1G; Net Carbs: 11G

Coconutty Cereal
Per Serving (Cereal Only):
Calories: 247; Total Fat: 24G;
Protein: 3G; Total Carbs: 7G;
Fiber: 6G; Net Carbs: 1G

Cinnamon "Sugar" Cereal
Calories: 405; Total Fat: 40G;
Protein: 4G; Total Carbs: 12G;
Fiber: 10G; Net Carbs: 2G

Keto Weight Loss Meal Plan without the Big 8 Allergens • WEEK 2

	MONDAY	TUESDAY	WEDNESDAY
MORNING	**Fatty Latte** Calories: 423; Total Fat: 47G; Protein: 2G; Total Carbs: 4G; Fiber: 1G; Net Carbs: 3G	**Fatty Latte** Calories: 423; Total Fat: 47G; Protein: 2G; Total Carbs: 4G; Fiber: 1G; Net Carbs: 3G	**Fatty Latte** Calories: 423; Total Fat: 47G; Protein: 2G; Total Carbs: 4G; Fiber: 1G; Net Carbs: 3G
MEAL 1	**Baked Dijon Chicken Legs** Calories: 316; Total Fat: 24G; Protein: 23G; Total Carbs: 2G; Fiber: 1G; Net Carbs: 1G **Mediterranean Wedge Salad** Calories: 196; Total Fat: 17G; Protein: 2G; Total Carbs: 12G; Fiber: 3G; Net Carbs: 9G	**Antipasto Salad** Calories: 240; Total Fat: 18G; Protein: 9G; Total Carbs: 14G; Fiber: 8G; Net Carbs: 6G	**Pork Burger Lettuce Cups** Calories: 395; Total Fat: 33G; Protein: 20G; Total Carbs: 5G; Fiber: 1G; Net Carbs: 4G
MEAL 2	**Sheet Pan Fajitas** Calories: 426; Total Fat: 30G; Protein: 26G; Total Carbs: 13G; Fiber: 3G; Net Carbs: 10G	**Vietnamese Steak and Cauliflower Rice Bowl** Calories: 466; Total Fat: 34G; Protein: 34G; Total Carbs: 6G; Fiber: 1G; Net Carbs: 5G	**Slow Cooker Chili With Bacon** Calories: 399; Total Fat: 27G; Protein: 30G; Total Carbs: 9G; Fiber: 1G; Net Carbs: 8G
DESSERT	**Fatty Hot Chocolate** Calories: 465; Total Fat: 49G; Protein: 6G; Total Carbs: 14G; Fiber: 3G; Net Carbs: 11G	**Blueberry-Coconut Smoothie** Calories: 506; Total Fat: 53G; Protein: 5G; Total Carbs: 12G; Fiber: 1G; Net Carbs: 11G	**Coconutty Cereal** Calories: 247; Total Fat: 24G; Protein: 3G; Total Carbs: 7G; Fiber: 6G; Net Carbs: 1G **Pink Passion Iced Tea** Calories: 114; Total Fat: 12G; Protein: 1G; Total Carbs: 2G; Fiber: 0G; Net Carbs: 2G
DRINK	3L water	3L water	3L water
TOTAL	Fat (167G)..............81.3% Protein (59G)...........12.9% Carbs (34G net).........5.8% Calories: 1826	Fat (152G)..............82.6% Protein (50G)...........12.2% Carbs (25G net).........5.2% Calories: 1635	Fat (143G)..............81.5% Protein (56G)...........14.2% Carbs (18G net).........4.3% Calories: 1578

+ Additional snack if desired

THURSDAY	FRIDAY	SATURDAY	SUNDAY
Fatty Latte Calories: 423; Total Fat: 47G; Protein: 2G; Total Carbs: 4G; Fiber: 1G; Net Carbs: 3G	**Fatty Latte** Calories: 423; Total Fat: 47G; Protein: 2G; Total Carbs: 4G; Fiber: 1G; Net Carbs: 3G	**Fatty Latte** Calories: 423; Total Fat: 47G; Protein: 2G; Total Carbs: 4G; Fiber: 1G; Net Carbs: 3G	**Fatty Latte** Calories: 423; Total Fat: 47G; Protein: 2G; Total Carbs: 4G; Fiber: 1G; Net Carbs: 3G
Chicken Coconut Curry Soup Calories: 410; Total Fat: 30G; Protein: 25G; Total Carbs: 10G; Fiber: 2G; Net Carbs: 8G	**Chopped Buffalo Chicken Salad** Calories: 336; Total Fat: 18G; Protein: 27G; Total Carbs: 21G; Fiber: 11G; Net Carbs: 10G **Bacon-Wrapped Asparagus** Calories: 244; Total Fat: 21G; Protein: 11G; Total Carbs: 3G; Fiber: 1G; Net Carbs: 2G	**Green Chile Meatballs** Calories: 326; Total Fat: 22G; Protein: 26G; Total Carbs: 6G; Fiber: 1G; Net Carbs: 5G **Mediterranean Wedge Salad** Calories: 196; Total Fat: 17G; Protein: 2G; Total Carbs: 12G; Fiber: 3G; Net Carbs: 9G	**Buttery Slow Cooker Pork Loin** Calories: 372; Total Fat: 19G; Protein: 47G; Total Carbs: 1G; Fiber: 0G; Net Carbs: 1G
Bacon-Wrapped Pork Nuggets Calories: 353; Total Fat: 30G; Protein: 20G; Total Carbs: 1G; Fiber: 0; Net Carbs: 1G **Buffalo Cauliflower** Calories: 145; Total Fat: 13G; Protein: 2G; Total Carbs: 5G; Fiber: 2G; Net Carbs: 3G	**Sriracha Pork Stir-Fry** Calories: 469; Total Fat: 38G; Protein: 24G; Total Carbs: 11G; Fiber: 4G; Net Carbs: 7G	**Oven-Baked Garlic and Herb Steak** Calories: 609; Total Fat: 48G; Protein: 36G; Total Carbs: 6G; Fiber: 2G; Net Carbs: 4G **Lemony Spinach** Calories: 82; Total Fat: 7G; Protein: 2G; Total Carbs: 4G; Fiber: 2G; Net Carbs: 2G	**Crispy Oven-Baked Pork Belly** Calories: 647; Total Fat: 67G; Protein: 11G; Total Carbs: 0G; Fiber: 0G; Net Carbs: 0G **Crispy Brussels Sprout Leaves** Calories: 49; Total Fat: 4G; Protein: 1G; Total Carbs: 4G; Fiber: 2G; Net Carbs: 2G
Fatty Hot Chocolate Calories: 465; Total Fat: 49G; Protein: 6G; Total Carbs: 14G; Fiber: 3G; Net Carbs: 11G			
3L water	3L water	3L water	3L water
Fat (169G) .... 82.7% Protein (55G) .... 12.3% Carbs (26G net) .... 5% Calories: 1795	Fat (124G) .... 75.8% Protein (64G) .... 17.4% Carbs (22G net) .... 6.8% Calories: 1472	Fat (141G) .... 77.6% Protein (78G) .... 18.1% Carbs (23G net).......... 4.3% Calories: 1636	Fat (137G) .... 81.6% Protein (61G) .... 15.3% Carbs (6G net) .... 3.1% Calories: 1491

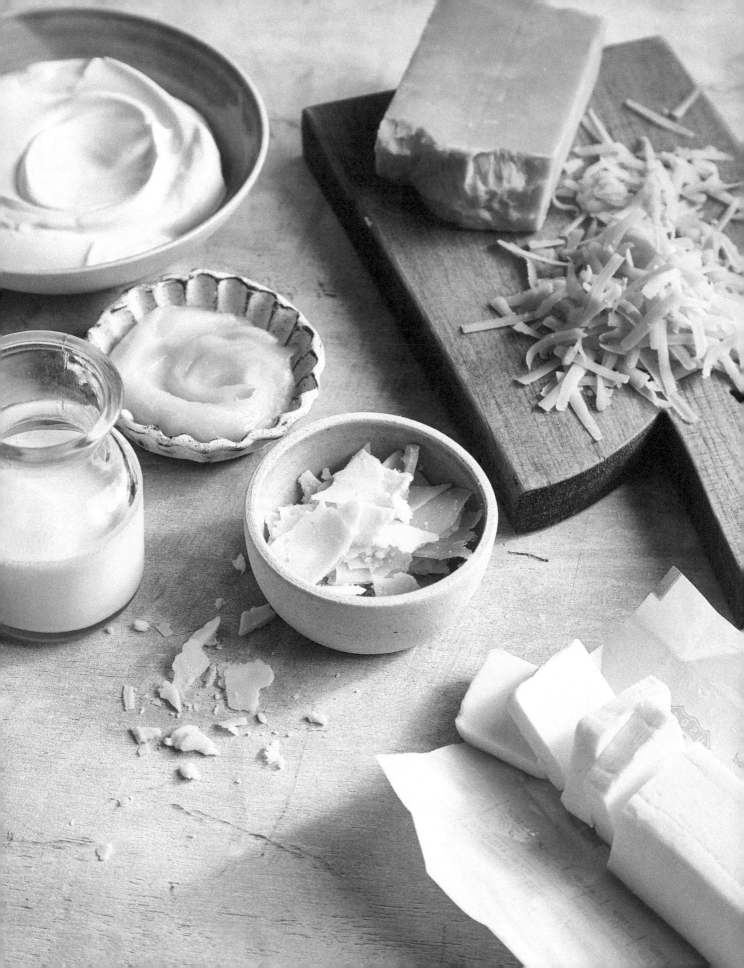

BASICS

CHAPTER THREE

HERBY BUTTER

PREP TIME: 5 MINUTES

An herb-filled butter melting over a nice juicy steak is one of the most incredible combinations. Making your own herby butter is simple, and you can use a mixture of whatever herbs you have on hand. *Serves 8*

○ COMFORT FOOD
● NUT-FREE
○ SUPER QUICK

8 ounces butter,
at room temperature

¼ teaspoon minced garlic

¼ cup chopped fresh herbs
(parsley, dill, and chives)

¼ teaspoon freshly ground
black pepper

1 teaspoon freshly squeezed
lemon juice

1. In a food processor or mixer, combine the butter, garlic, herbs, pepper, and lemon juice.

2. Mix thoroughly for about a minute, but don't whip.

Variation: Rosemary, thyme, and sage is also a great combination.

MACRONUTRIENTS	99.5% FAT	0.5% PROTEIN	0% CARBS

CALORIES: 202; TOTAL FAT: 23G; PROTEIN: 0G; TOTAL CARBS: 0G; FIBER: 0G; NET CARBS: 0G

BEEF BONE BROTH

PREP TIME: 15 MINUTES **COOK TIME:** 9 TO 25 HOURS

Bone broth is incredibly good for your gut and is super nourishing. The longer you cook the broth, the more concentrated and full of collagen it will be. You can sip the broth alone, or you can use it as a base for a soup. Be sure to blanch and roast the bones to remove impurities and to caramelize the bones to add flavor and depth to the finished broth. For the best selection, visit your butcher and get joint bones like cow knuckles and neck bones. *Serves 6*

● ALLERGEN-FREE
○ COMFORT FOOD
◐ DAIRY-FREE
● NUT-FREE
● PALEO OR PALEO-FRIENDLY

4 pounds beef bones

1 onion, quartered

1 garlic head, cut horizontally

2 tablespoons freshly ground black pepper

1. In a large pot, cover the bones with cold water and bring to a boil over high heat for 20 minutes. Drain.

2. Preheat the oven to 450°F.

3. On a large baking sheet, arrange the bones in a single layer and cook for 45 minutes.

4. Transfer the bones, along with any crispy bits on the baking sheet, to the large pot.

5. Add the onion, garlic, and pepper.

6. Add just enough water to cover the bones. Bring to a boil, lower the heat, and cover.

7. Bone broth should simmer for as long as possible, about 8 hours minimum, but ideally up to 24 hours.

8. Remove the pot from the heat and let it cool slightly. Strain the broth with a mesh sieve, discarding the bones and vegetables.

9. Let the broth continue to cool until barely warm and transfer to smaller containers to store in the refrigerator or freezer.

Make Ahead: Bone broth can be stored in the refrigerator for 5 days or in the freezer for up to 6 months.

MACRONUTRIENTS	40% FAT	57% PROTEIN	3% CARBS

CALORIES: 194; TOTAL FAT: 9G; PROTEIN: 27G; TOTAL CARBS: 2G; FIBER: 1G; NET CARBS: 1G

BACON

PREP TIME: 5 MINUTES **COOK TIME:** 20 MINUTES

I love to bake my bacon! It makes it easy to make larger amounts at once and keeps my stove top clean. You can bake whole slices or cut them into smaller "chips." Either way works great. *Serves 4*

● ALLERGEN-FREE
○ COMFORT FOOD
◐ DAIRY-FREE
● NUT-FREE
● PALEO OR PALEO-FRIENDLY
○ SUPER QUICK

1 pound bacon, uncured

1. Preheat the oven to 400°F.

2. Line a large baking sheet with aluminum foil all the way to the edges. You can use a rack on top of the foil if you want to, but I put the bacon right on the foil.

3. On the prepared baking sheet, arrange the bacon in a single layer, with a little overlapping if needed.

4. Bake for 20 minutes on the middle rack of the oven, until the bacon reaches your desired crispiness.

5. Transfer the bacon to a paper towel–lined plate to soak up any excess grease.

Variation: Have you ever sprinkled Parmesan cheese, garlic powder, and fresh parsley on your bacon? It's delicious. To try it, pull the bacon out after 10 minutes, sprinkle those three ingredients on top, and cook for 10 more minutes.

MACRONUTRIENTS	71% FAT	28% PROTEIN	1% CARBS

CALORIES: 173; TOTAL FAT: 13G; PROTEIN: 12G; TOTAL CARBS: 0G; FIBER: 0G; NET CARBS: 0G

SAUSAGE PATTIES

PREP TIME: 5 MINUTES **COOK TIME:** 10 MINUTES

I like to know what is in my food whenever possible. I just don't trust prepared sausage patties that you can buy at the store, so I make my own. Luckily it's super simple, and you can tailor the seasoning to your liking. If you like extra flavor, you can replace ground pork with ground chorizo instead. *Serves 4*

● ALLERGEN-FREE
○ COMFORT FOOD
◐ DAIRY-FREE
● NUT-FREE
● PALEO OR PALEO-FRIENDLY
○ SUPER QUICK

½ pound ground pork

1 teaspoon garlic powder

¼ teaspoon red pepper flakes

½ teaspoon fennel seeds

Salt

Freshly ground black pepper

1 tablespoon extra-virgin olive oil

1. In a medium bowl, mix the ground pork, garlic powder, red pepper flakes, and fennel seeds. Season with salt and pepper.

2. Using your hands, form the mixture into 4 patties.

3. In a skillet, heat the olive oil over medium-high heat.

4. Cook the sausage patties for 5 minutes on each side, flipping once, until cooked through.

5. Transfer the sausage patties to a paper towel–lined plate to soak up any excess grease.

Make Ahead: You can freeze these sausage patties for up to 6 months.

MACRONUTRIENTS	76% FAT	23% PROTEIN	1% CARBS

CALORIES: 182; TOTAL FAT: 15G; PROTEIN: 10G; TOTAL CARBS: 1G; FIBER: 0G; NET CARBS: 1G

BAKED AVOCADO

PREP TIME: 5 MINUTES **COOK TIME:** 30 MINUTES

Baked avocados are a great way to make a quick, easy meal with just a few ingredients you probably already have in your refrigerator or pantry. You'll want to scoop out some of the avocado meat to make room for the egg in this recipe. Consider it a snack while you wait for the rest of the dish to bake! *Serves 2*

○ COMFORT FOOD
◐ DAIRY-FREE
● NUT-FREE
● PALEO OR PALEO-FRIENDLY

1 avocado, halved and pitted

1 teaspoon Tajín sauce (optional)

2 large eggs

Salt

Freshly ground black pepper

1. Preheat the oven to 350°F.

2. Use a melon baller to scoop out 1 tablespoon or so of avocado flesh from each half to make more space for the eggs.

3. Sprinkle the avocado with the Tajín sauce (if using) for an extra kick.

4. On a baking sheet or muffin tin, place both avocado halves with the cut sides up.

5. Crack 1 egg into each side of the avocado and season with salt and pepper.

6. Bake for 25 to 30 minutes, depending on how you like your egg cooked. Serve.

Variation: The egg and avocado is a delicious combination on its own, but you can also top it with crumbled bacon, Parmesan cheese, or Pico de Gallo (page 250) for fun variations.

MACRONUTRIENTS	72% FAT	16% PROTEIN	12% CARBS

CALORIES: 185; TOTAL FAT: 15G; PROTEIN: 8G; TOTAL CARBS: 6G; FIBER: 5G; NET CARBS: 1G

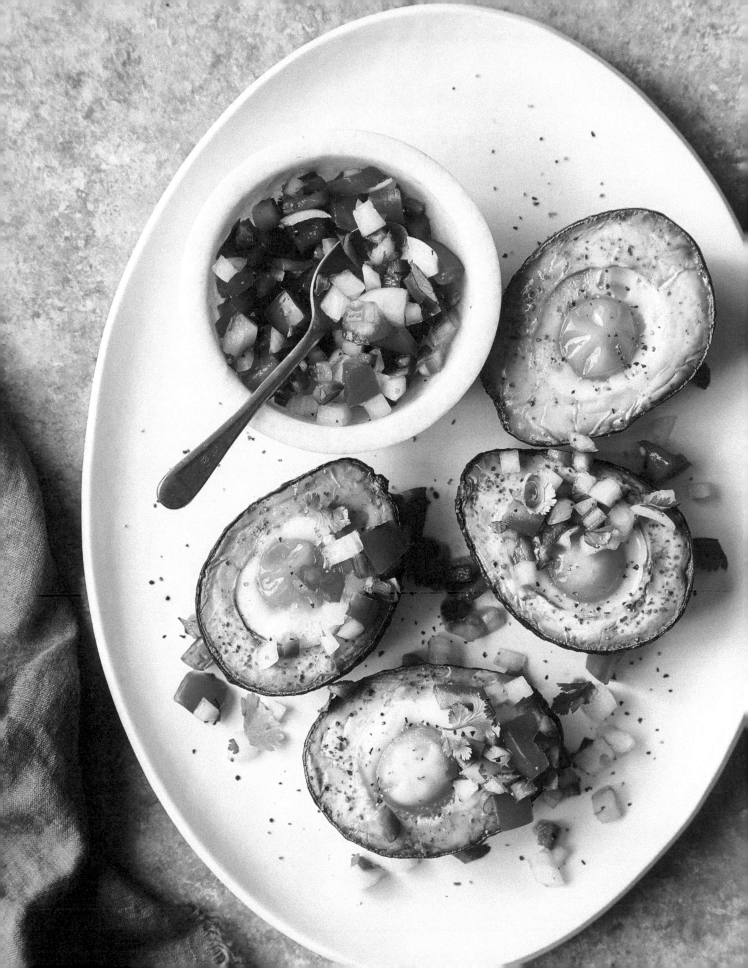

CAULIFLOWER RICE

PREP TIME: 5 MINUTES **COOK TIME:** 10 MINUTES

Cauliflower is one of the most versatile ingredients on the planet and is used in many, many ways within the keto diet. Cauliflower rice will allow you to create all of your favorite rice dishes, but keto-fied. *Serves 2*

- ● ALLERGEN-FREE
- ○ COMFORT FOOD
- ◐ DAIRY-FREE
- ● NUT-FREE
- ● PALEO OR PALEO-FRIENDLY
- ○ SUPER QUICK

2 tablespoons extra-virgin olive oil

½ small onion, diced

½ cauliflower head

Salt

Freshly ground black pepper

2 tablespoons chopped fresh parsley

1. In a skillet, heat the olive oil over medium-high heat.

2. Add the onion and cook for about 5 minutes, until softened.

3. While the onion is cooking, cut the cauliflower head into florets, discarding the stem.

4. In a food processor, pulse the cauliflower until it resembles rice.

5. Add the cauliflower to the skillet, season with salt and pepper, and stir frequently. Cook for 5 minutes, or for as long as 10 minutes if you like it crispy.

6. Once the cauliflower rice is finished, divide into bowls and top with the parsley.

Variation: Cauliflower rice can take on a huge variety of flavors, so use this recipe as a base and get creative. Creamy garlic, cilantro lime, Spanish seasonings, Indian seasonings, or a new take on fried rice are all great variations.

MACRONUTRIENTS	67% FAT	6% PROTEIN	27% CARBS

CALORIES: 180; TOTAL FAT: 14G; PROTEIN: 4G; TOTAL CARBS: 13G; FIBER: 6G; NET CARBS: 7G

ZOODLES (SPIRALIZED ZUCCHINI NOODLES)

PREP TIME: 5 MINUTES **COOK TIME:** 5 MINUTES

Zoodles (spiralized zucchini noodles) are a great way to turn high-carb noodle dishes into low-carb keto dishes. Zucchini is the most common vegetable used for keto dishes because other frequently used vegetables like sweet potatoes are not keto-friendly. There are various spiralizer tools available. Personally, whenever I see prespiralized zoodles at the grocery store, I pick up a pack. You can eat the zoodles raw in cold dishes or cooked in a skillet. *Serves 2*

● ALLERGEN-FREE
○ COMFORT FOOD
◐ DAIRY-FREE
● NUT-FREE
● PALEO OR PALEO-FRIENDLY
○ SUPER QUICK

1 tablespoon extra-virgin olive oil

1 garlic clove, minced

2 zucchini, spiralized

Salt

Freshly ground black pepper

1. In a skillet, heat the olive oil over medium heat.

2. Add the garlic and sauté for 30 seconds, then add the zoodles and toss.

3. Cook for 2 to 3 minutes, stirring throughout.

4. Season the zoodles with salt and pepper. Toss in sauce if desired.

Variation: Zoodles Alfredo is my go-to dinner when I have a protein-filled lunch and need to go lighter for dinner. It is delicious!

MACRONUTRIENTS	71% FAT	10% PROTEIN	19% CARBS

CALORIES: 91; TOTAL FAT: 7G; PROTEIN: 4G; TOTAL CARBS: 5G; FIBER: 2G; NET CARBS: 3G

ROASTED VEGGIES

PREP TIME: 5 MINUTES **COOK TIME:** 20 TO 25 MINUTES

You can roast pretty much any vegetable! Roasting is my absolute favorite way to eat veggies such as cauliflower, broccoli, and Brussels sprouts. Just make sure you chop the vegetables into pieces that are about the same size so that they roast evenly. *Serves 4*

○ ALLERGEN-FREE
○ COMFORT FOOD
◦ DAIRY-FREE
● NUT-FREE
● PALEO OR PALEO-FRIENDLY
○ SUPER QUICK

1 cup cauliflower florets

1 cup broccoli florets

1 cup Brussels sprouts

2 tablespoons extra-virgin olive oil

Salt

Freshly ground black pepper

1. Preheat the oven to 425°F.

2. In a medium bowl, toss the cauliflower, broccoli, and Brussels sprouts with olive oil, and season with salt and pepper.

3. On a baking sheet, spread the vegetables in a single layer. Be careful not to crowd them or the vegetables might steam rather than roast.

4. Cook the vegetables for 20 to 25 minutes, stirring once about halfway through.

5. Sprinkle with a little more salt and pepper before serving.

Variation: Another great mix of vegetables is green beans, zucchini, asparagus, and bell peppers. This mix needs to roast for only about 15 minutes—otherwise prepare the same way.

MACRONUTRIENTS	74% FAT	6% PROTEIN	20% CARBS

CALORIES: 83; TOTAL FAT: 7G; PROTEIN: 2G; TOTAL CARBS: 5G; FIBER: 2G; NET CARBS: 3G

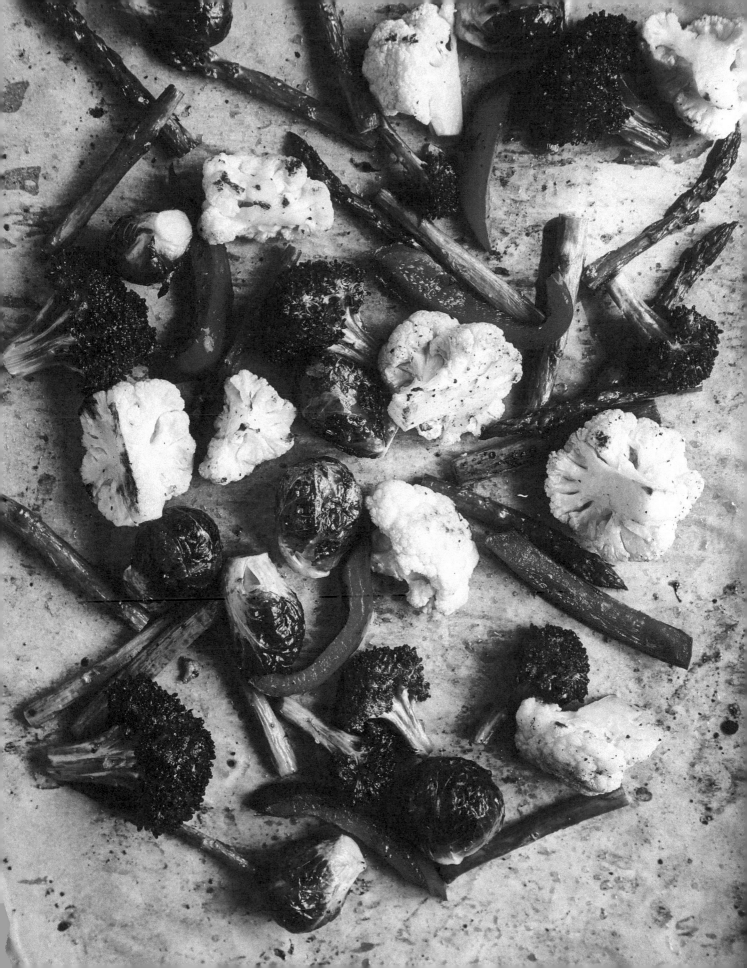

SHIRATAKI NOODLES

PREP TIME: 5 MINUTES **COOK TIME:** 7 MINUTES

Shirataki noodles are made with a fiber-packed glucomannan starch and have zero net carbs and zero calories. They are light and allow you to create all of your favorite pasta dishes, but without the carbs. The key is to make sure you follow the instructions because the cooking directions are very different from those of wheat pasta. *Serves 2*

● ALLERGEN-FREE
○ COMFORT FOOD
◉ DAIRY-FREE
● NUT-FREE
● PALEO OR PALEO-FRIENDLY
○ SUPER QUICK

1 (7-ounce) package shirataki noodles (or shirataki rice)

1. Fill a saucepan about halfway with water and bring to a boil over high heat.

2. Rinse the shirataki noodles under cold water for 30 seconds in a colander.

3. Add the noodles to the boiling water and cook for 2 minutes.

4. Transfer the noodles to a dry skillet on medium heat and cook for 3 to 5 minutes to dry them out until they are opaque.

Variation: Once the noodles are cooked, they can be added to any sauce or broth.

MACRONUTRIENTS	0% FAT	0% PROTEIN	100% CARBS

CALORIES: 2; TOTAL FAT: 0G; PROTEIN: 0G; TOTAL CARBS: 0.5G; FIBER: 0.5G; NET CARBS: 0G

KETO PUMPKIN BREAD

PREP TIME: 5 MINUTES **COOK TIME:** 25 MINUTES

I love baking this bread. The taste of pumpkin reminds me of fall no matter what time of year it is. You can also make great French toast with thicker slices. *Serves 12*

○ COMFORT FOOD
○ SUPER QUICK

Butter, shortening, or lard, for greasing

6 large eggs

4 tablespoons butter, at room temperature

¼ cup pumpkin purée (not pumpkin pie mix)

3 teaspoons erythritol

1 tablespoon pumpkin pie spice

1½ cups almond flour

3 teaspoons baking powder

1 scoop MCT oil powder (optional)

Pinch salt

1. Preheat the oven to 390°F.

2. Grease a loaf pan with butter, shortening, or lard.

3. In a mixer bowl, combine the eggs, butter, pumpkin purée, erythritol, pumpkin pie spice, almond flour, baking powder, MCT oil powder (if using), and a pinch of salt. Blend until smooth.

4. Pour the mixture into the prepared pan and bake for 25 minutes, until a toothpick inserted in the bread comes out clean.

Variation: You can make your own pumpkin pie spice mix with a combination of cinnamon, nutmeg, ginger, and allspice.

| MACRONUTRIENTS | 77% FAT | 17% PROTEIN | 0% CARBS |

CALORIES: 90; TOTAL FAT: 8G; PROTEIN: 4G; TOTAL CARBS: 1G; FIBER: 0G; NET CARBS: 1G; ERYTHRITOL: 1G

CLOUD OOPSIE ROLLS

PREP TIME: 20 MINUTES **COOK TIME:** 35 MINUTES

Oopsie rolls are a staple of keto recipe lists, and if you are craving bread or a sandwich, this is a great way to go. They are very low in carbs and high in fat, which fits in perfectly with keto macros. The cream of tartar makes the rolls nice and fluffy, so be sure not to leave that out. *Serves 8*

○ COMFORT FOOD
● NUT-FREE

2 large eggs

⅛ teaspoon cream of tartar

2 ounces cream cheese, cubed

Pinch salt

1. Preheat the oven to 300°F. Line a baking sheet with parchment paper or a silicone mat.

2. Separate the egg yolks and whites.

3. Using a mixer, beat the egg whites until bubbly. Add the cream of tartar and beat into stiff peaks.

4. In a separate bowl, beat together the egg yolks, cream cheese, and salt. The yolks will become pale yellow once fully mixed.

5. Using a rubber scraper, fold the egg whites into the yolk mixture.

6. Spoon hamburger bun–size dollops onto the sheet.

7. Bake for 35 minutes, until the rolls are golden and firm.

8. Allow the rolls to cool; once cooled they can be stored in an airtight container and refrigerated for about a week.

Variation: You can add vanilla extract and erythritol to this recipe to create easy, individual serving–size keto-friendly cakes.

MACRONUTRIENTS	77% FAT	19% PROTEIN	4% CARBS

CALORIES: 42; TOTAL FAT: 4G; PROTEIN: 2G; TOTAL CARBS: 0G; FIBER: 0G; NET CARBS: 0G

KETO CREAM CHEESE "FLUFF"

PREP TIME: 5 MINUTES

Keto "Fluff" is a super-simple dessert. I have been known to eat whipped cream cheese with a spoon, and this recipe takes that concept one step further by adding a depth of flavor with the vanilla and erythritol. *Serves 2*

○ COMFORT FOOD
● NUT-FREE
○ SUPER QUICK

4 ounces cream cheese, cubed

1 tablespoon heavy whipping cream

1 teaspoon erythritol

1 teaspoon vanilla extract

In a food processor, combine the cream cheese, cream, erythritol, and vanilla, and process until smooth. Eat immediately or chill before serving.

Variation: There are tons of ways to customize this base. You can blend in berries for a fresh addition. You can also blend in sugar-free syrups or use different extracts.

MACRONUTRIENTS	89% FAT	9% PROTEIN	2% CARBS

CALORIES: 219; TOTAL FAT: 22G; PROTEIN: 3G; TOTAL CARBS: 1G; FIBER: 0G; NET CARBS: 1G; ERYTHRITOL: 2G

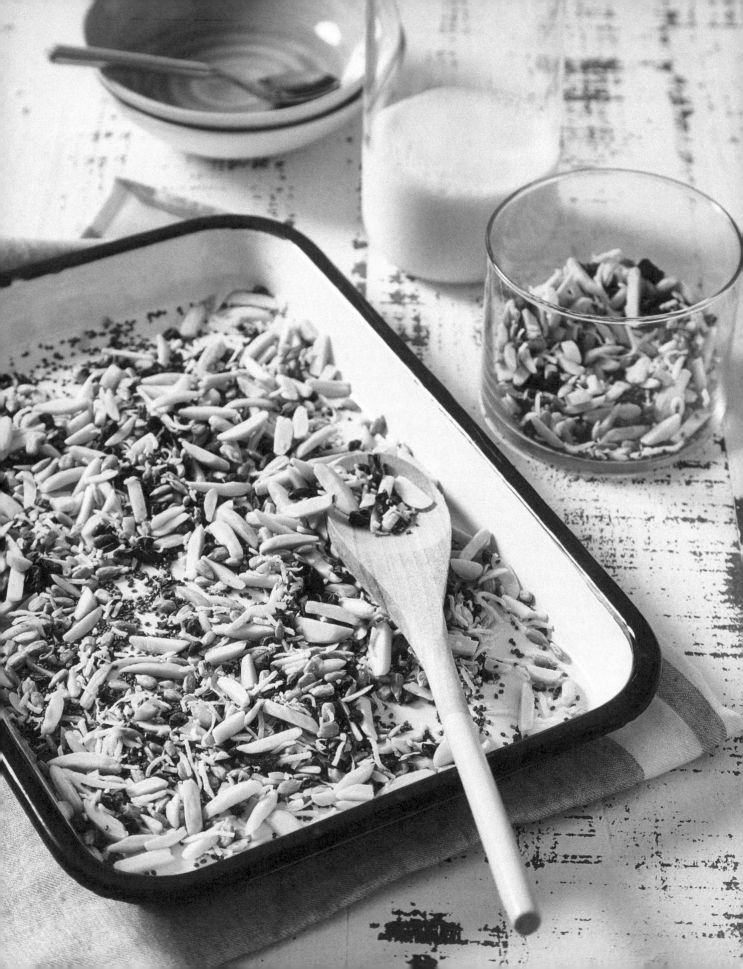

DAIRY AND NUTS

CHAPTER FOUR

Opposite: Cacao Crunch Cereal

SPICY PECANS

PREP TIME: 5 MINUTES **COOK TIME:** 5 MINUTES

Nuts are a great snack that is full of healthy fats. You can add a lot of great flavors in just minutes in the skillet. I prefer to make my own seasoned nuts because it's quick and easy, and I know exactly what the ingredients are. It is also fun to try new combinations! *Serves 4*

○ DAIRY-FREE

● PALEO OR PALEO-FRIENDLY

○ SUPER QUICK

1 teaspoon ground cumin

1 teaspoon chili powder

Salt

Freshly ground black pepper

2 cups pecans

1 tablespoon extra-virgin olive oil or ghee

1. In a medium bowl, mix the cumin, chili powder, salt, and pepper.

2. Heat a dry skillet over medium heat. Once hot, add the pecans and toast for about 5 minutes, until lightly browned.

3. Transfer the browned nuts into the bowl with the seasoning mixture, add the olive oil, and mix until the nuts are coated.

4. Pour the nuts onto a baking sheet lined with parchment paper or a silicone baking mat to cool.

Variation: You can substitute or add other nuts to this mixture, like almonds or walnuts.

MACRONUTRIENTS	88% FAT	4% PROTEIN	8% CARBS

CALORIES: 375; TOTAL FAT: 39G; PROTEIN: 5G; TOTAL CARBS: 7G; FIBER: 5G; NET CARBS: 2G

CINNAMON ROASTED ALMONDS

PREP TIME: 5 MINUTES **COOK TIME:** 5 MINUTES

Cinnamon is one of those ingredients that are delicious and also have lots of health benefits, like being anti-inflammatory. I love this simple recipe for adding cinnamon to almonds, and if you are feeling like something sweet, you can also add a teaspoon of erythritol to the mix. *Serves 4*

DAIRY-FREE

● PALEO OR PALEO-FRIENDLY

○ SUPER QUICK

1 teaspoon ground cinnamon

Salt

2 cups almonds

1 tablespoon extra-virgin olive oil or ghee

1. In a medium bowl, mix the cinnamon and salt.

2. Heat a dry skillet over medium heat. Once hot, add the almonds and toast for about 5 minutes, until browned.

3. Transfer the almonds to the bowl with the cinnamon mixture, add the olive oil, and mix until the nuts are coated.

4. Pour the nuts onto a baking sheet lined with parchment paper or a silicone baking mat to cool.

Variation: You can also roast these in the oven for 1 hour at 250°F.

MACRONUTRIENTS	74% FAT	12% PROTEIN	14% CARBS

CALORIES: 453; TOTAL FAT: 40G; PROTEIN: 16G; TOTAL CARBS: 15G; FIBER: 8G; NET CARBS: 7G

CACAO CRUNCH CEREAL

PREP TIME: 5 MINUTES

Craving cereal without all of the sugar? This healthy combination will give you the crunch and sweetness while also being loaded with fiber and healthy fats. I don't add erythritol, but you can if you prefer—or you can add a couple of berries for natural sweetness. Strawberries and cacao nibs is a delicious combination! *Serves 2*

○ DAIRY-FREE

● PALEO OR PALEO-FRIENDLY

○ SUPER QUICK

½ cup slivered almonds

2 tablespoons coconut, shredded or flakes

2 tablespoons chia seeds

2 tablespoons cacao nibs

2 tablespoons sunflower seeds

Unsweetened nondairy milk of choice (I use macadamia milk), for serving

1. In a small bowl, combine the almonds, coconut, chia seeds, cacao nibs, and sunflower seeds. Divide between two bowls.

2. Pour in the nondairy milk and serve.

MACRONUTRIENTS	70% FAT	11% PROTEIN	19% CARBS

PER SERVING (CEREAL ONLY): CALORIES: 325; TOTAL FAT: 27; PROTEIN: 10G; TOTAL CARBS: 17G; FIBER: 12G; NET CARBS: 5G

COCONUTTY CEREAL

PREP TIME: 5 MINUTES **COOK TIME:** 5 MINUTES

This cereal is so simple, but toasting the coconut flakes gives it a great crunch with a hint of sweetness that will trick you into thinking you are eating a high-carb cereal. *Serves 2*

DAIRY-FREE
SUPER QUICK

1 cup coconut, shredded or flakes

1 teaspoon erythritol

Unsweetened nondairy milk of choice (I use macadamia milk), for serving

1. Preheat the oven to 350°F.

2. On a baking sheet, arrange the coconut flakes in a single layer.

3. Bake for about 5 minutes, until nice and golden.

4. Let the coconut flakes cool for 5 to 10 minutes, then toss them with the erythritol in a plastic ziptop bag and shake.

5. Divide between two bowls and pour in the nondairy milk. Serve.

Variation: You can add berries for additional natural sweetness.

MACRONUTRIENTS	87% FAT	5% PROTEIN	8% CARBS

CALORIES: 247; TOTAL FAT: 24G; PROTEIN: 3G; TOTAL CARBS: 7G; FIBER: 6G; NET CARBS: 1G; ERYTHRITOL: 2G

CINNAMON "SUGAR" CEREAL

PREP TIME: 5 MINUTES **COOK TIME:** 10 MINUTES

You know that one brand of sugar-filled cereal that tastes like crispy French toast? This recipe is my keto-fied version. I love the cinnamon, and the cacao nibs make it extra special. The nondairy milk you choose will also help enhance the flavors in different ways, so don't be afraid to try new ones—just make sure you buy unsweetened. *Serves 2*

○ DAIRY-FREE
○ SUPER QUICK

1 cup coconut, shredded or flakes

2 tablespoons butter or ghee

1 tablespoon ground cinnamon

1 teaspoon erythritol

2 tablespoons cacao nibs

Unsweetened nondairy milk of choice (I use macadamia milk), for serving

1. Preheat the oven to 325°F.

2. Place the coconut flakes in a small bowl.

3. In a saucepan, add the butter, cinnamon, and erythritol over medium heat, melt, and mix well.

4. Pour the mixture over the coconut flakes, stir to mix, and then lay the coated coconut flakes on the baking sheet in a single layer.

5. Bake for 5 to 7 minutes, or until nice and golden. Stir the coconut flakes a couple of times to toast all sides and make sure they don't burn.

6. Let the coconut flakes cool for 5 to 10 minutes.

7. Divide between two bowls, add the cacao nibs, and pour in the nondairy milk to serve.

Make Ahead: You can make a larger portion of this and store it in an airtight container in the refrigerator for up to a week.

MACRONUTRIENTS	84% FAT	4% PROTEIN	12% CARBS

CALORIES: 405; TOTAL FAT: 40G; PROTEIN: 4G; TOTAL CARBS: 12G; FIBER: 10G; NET CARBS: 2G; ERYTHRITOL: 2G

CRUNCHY GRANOLA

PREP TIME: 5 MINUTES **COOK TIME:** 25 MINUTES

It is so easy to make your own granola. If you're like me, you have a bunch of nuts and seeds in the house anyway, so combine them and create something delicious! This makes a great snack or breakfast on the go—plus it's so simple that you can have your kids help make it. (I've always found that kids are a lot more likely to eat something they had a part in creating!) *Serves 4*

○ DAIRY-FREE
● PALEO-FRIENDLY
○ SUPER QUICK

1 cup mixed nuts
(pecans, pilis, macadamias, walnuts, almonds, hazelnuts)

½ cup mixed seeds
(flaxseed, sunflower seeds, pumpkin seeds, chia seeds)

½ cup coconut, shredded or flakes

¼ cup almond flour

1 tablespoon erythritol

Pinch salt

2 tablespoons butter or ghee, melted

1 large egg

2 tablespoons cacao nibs

1. Preheat the oven to 325°F. Line a baking sheet with parchment paper and set aside.

2. In a food processor, pulse the nuts a couple of times to break them down slightly, keeping some good-size chunks.

3. In a medium bowl, toss the chopped nuts, seeds, coconut flakes, almond flour, and erythritol. Season with salt. Stir and then mix in the butter and egg.

4. Spread the mixture onto the prepared baking sheet and sprinkle the cacao nibs on top.

5. Bake for 25 minutes, stirring every 5 to 10 minutes to get all sides golden brown.

Make It Paleo: Omit the erythritol.

| MACRONUTRIENTS | 84% FAT | 9% PROTEIN | 7% CARBS |

CALORIES: 432; TOTAL FAT: 43G; PROTEIN: 8G; TOTAL CARBS: 8G; FIBER: 7G; NET CARBS: 1G; ERYTHRITOL: 3G

MACADAMIA NUT SQUARES

PREP TIME: 10 MINUTES, PLUS 1 HOUR TO CHILL

Macadamia nuts are my favorite, so I loved the idea of combining them with nut butter to create a treat that works for breakfast or as a dessert. I use Legendary Foods Apple Pie Almond & Cashew Butter with this recipe, but you can use any nut butter you wish. Use a loaf pan, or if you don't have one, make a double batch and use a 9-by-9-inch baking dish. *Serves 4*

¼ cup macadamia nuts

¼ cup nut butter

1 teaspoon erythritol

2 tablespoons butter, melted

2 tablespoons shredded coconut or cacao nibs (optional)

1. In a food processor, pulse the macadamia nuts until they are a little smaller than rice size.

2. In a bowl, combine the macadamia nuts, nut butter, erythritol, and butter and mix well. Add the shredded coconut and/or cacao nibs (if using) and stir well.

3. Line a loaf pan with parchment paper and pour the mixture into the pan.

4. Refrigerate for 1 hour, remove, and cut into squares. Store in an airtight container, refrigerated or in the freezer.

Variation: There are some great keto-friendly nut butters out there—experiment to create your own flavor combinations. Or find a brand that makes unique flavors. One of my favorite brands makes flavors like blueberry cinnamon roll, pecan pie, and apple pie.

MACRONUTRIENTS	87% FAT	7% PROTEIN	6% CARBS

CALORIES: 208; TOTAL FAT: 21G; PROTEIN: 3G; TOTAL CARBS: 3G; FIBER: 1G; NET CARBS: 2G; ERYTHRITOL: 1G

BERRY CHEESECAKE BARS

PREP TIME: 10 MINUTES **COOK TIME:** 25 MINUTES

Berries and cheesecake are pretty much all I need in life to be happy, so this dairy-filled bar is heaven for me. It is very simple, and the cheesecake base is easy to customize with other flavors. Make this in a small casserole or loaf pan, or if desired, use a well-greased muffin tin to make individual cheesecakes. *Serves 4*

○ COMFORT FOOD
● NUT-FREE

4 tablespoons butter, melted

2 large eggs

4 tablespoons cream cheese

1 teaspoon vanilla extract

¼ teaspoon baking powder

1 to 2 tablespoons confectioners' erythritol

2 tablespoons frozen blueberries or mixed berries

1. Preheat the oven to 325°F.

2. In a medium bowl, combine the butter, eggs, cream cheese, vanilla, baking powder, and erythritol.

3. Using a hand mixer or an immersion blender, mix thoroughly until completely smooth.

4. Line a small casserole or loaf pan with parchment paper and pour the mixture into it.

5. Drop the blueberries in last, distributing them evenly so you get some in every bar. They will sink as they cook, so do not mix.

6. Bake for 20 to 25 minutes, until just set but still with a little jiggle.

7. Cool completely, flip the dish upside down, cut into bars, and serve.

Variation: I use confectioners' erythritol in this recipe, but you can use granulated erythritol if that is all you have.

MACRONUTRIENTS	88% FAT	9% PROTEIN	3% CARBS

CALORIES: 189; TOTAL FAT: 19G; PROTEIN: 4G; TOTAL CARBS: 2G; FIBER: 0G; NET CARBS: 2G; ERYTHRITOL: 3G

CHOCOLATE DRIZZLE MACADAMIA BREAKFAST COOKIES

PREP TIME: 10 MINUTES **COOK TIME:** 12 MINUTES

Who doesn't love cookies for breakfast? It feels so naughty, but these cookies kick your day off with healthy fats that will keep you full for hours. I love the chewy texture. Pop them in the refrigerator and have a decadent breakfast ready for the whole week. *Serves 8*

○ **COMFORT FOOD**
○ **SUPER QUICK**

4 tablespoons unsalted butter

1¼ cups almond flour

¼ cup erythritol

¼ teaspoon salt

¼ teaspoon cream of tartar

1 large egg

1 teaspoon vanilla extract

¼ cup chopped macadamia nuts or nuts of choice

¼ cup sugar-free chocolate chips

1. Preheat the oven to 350°F. Line a baking sheet with parchment paper or a silicone mat and set aside.

2. In a saucepan, melt the butter over low heat. Transfer the butter to a small bowl and place in the refrigerator for 10 minutes to cool down.

3. In a large bowl, combine the almond flour, erythritol, salt, and cream of tartar. Stir to combine.

4. In another small bowl, combine the egg, vanilla, and cooled butter. Whisk together.

5. Pour the wet ingredients into the dry ingredients and combine everything together with a large spoon or rubber scraper. Fold in the macadamia nuts.

MACRONUTRIENTS	88% FAT	7% PROTEIN	5% CARBS

CALORIES: 156; TOTAL FAT: 12G; PROTEIN: 3G; TOTAL CARBS: 7G; FIBER: 1G; NET CARBS: 6G; ERYTHRITOL: 2G

6. Scoop out 2-inch balls of cookie dough and arrange them on the prepared baking sheet. I like to flatten mine a bit.

7. Bake the cookies for 10 to 12 minutes, until the edges are golden brown.

8. Let the cookies rest for 10 to 15 minutes before transferring them to a cooling rack. Cool for an additional 15 minutes.

9. Melt the chocolate in the microwave for 30 seconds at 50 percent power. Stir and heat in small increments until melted.

10. Using a rubber scraper dipped in melted chocolate, drizzle the chocolate over the cookies. Transfer the cookies to the refrigerator to set.

Make Ahead: These cookies will keep for a week in the refrigerator.

CREAM CHEESE BLUEBERRY MUFFINS

PREP TIME: 10 MINUTES **COOK TIME:** 12 MINUTES

Blueberry muffins are an ultimate comfort food for me. When I was a teenager, I used to make the boxed variety all the time, so blueberry muffins really bring me back. Now I make this keto-friendly version, and they are even more delicious. I slather them with butter before eating, and they are so good! *Serves 6*

○ **COMFORT FOOD**
○ **SUPER QUICK**

Nonstick cooking spray

1 cup almond flour

2 teaspoons ground cinnamon

3 to 4 tablespoons erythritol

¾ tablespoon baking powder

2 large eggs

2 tablespoons cream cheese

2 tablespoons heavy whipping cream

4 tablespoons butter, melted and cooled

2 teaspoons vanilla extract

2 tablespoons blueberries (fresh or frozen)

1. Preheat the oven to 400°F. Spray a muffin tin with cooking spray or line it with muffin liners.

2. In a small bowl, mix the almond flour, cinnamon, erythritol, and baking powder.

3. In a medium bowl, mix the eggs, cream cheese, heavy cream, butter, and vanilla with a hand mixer.

4. Pour the flour mixture into the egg mixture and beat with the hand mixer until thoroughly mixed.

5. Pour the mixture into the prepared muffin cups.

6. Drop the berries on top of the batter in the muffin cups.

7. Bake for 12 minutes, or until golden brown on top, and serve.

Variation: You can also replace the cream cheese–heavy whipping cream combination with ½ cup of sour cream.

MACRONUTRIENTS	85% FAT	9% PROTEIN	6% CARBS

CALORIES: 160; TOTAL FAT: 15G; PROTEIN: 4G; TOTAL CARBS: 10G; FIBER: 2G; NET CARBS: 8G

PUMPKIN SPICE PANCAKES

PREP TIME: 5 MINUTES **COOK TIME:** 10 MINUTES

I love to make these pancakes when I have a little pumpkin left over—sometimes from making Keto Pumpkin Bread (page 41). Add some vanilla and a warm spice like cinnamon for a yummy combination. *Serves 6*

○ COMFORT FOOD
● NUT-FREE
○ SUPER QUICK

2 tablespoons pumpkin purée
(not pumpkin pie mix)

4 large eggs

4 ounces cream cheese,
at room temperature

1 teaspoon erythritol

2 teaspoons ground cinnamon
or pumpkin pie spice

4 tablespoons coconut flour

2 teaspoons vanilla extract

1½ teaspoons baking powder

4 tablespoons butter, divided

1. In a food processor, mix the pumpkin purée, eggs, cream cheese, erythritol, cinnamon, coconut flour, vanilla, and baking powder. Thoroughly combine until you have a smooth consistency.

2. In a large skillet over medium-high heat, melt 2 tablespoons of butter.

3. Pour the batter into the skillet in ¼-cup portions.

4. The pancakes will get puffy when it is time to flip them, after about 2 minutes. Cook for about 1 minute on the other side, or until lightly browned.

5. Repeat with the remaining 2 tablespoons of butter for the remaining batter.

Make Ahead: These reheat well, so make a double batch and have pancakes all week.

MACRONUTRIENTS	85% FAT	9% PROTEIN	6% CARBS

CALORIES: 160; TOTAL FAT: 15G; PROTEIN: 4G; TOTAL CARBS: 8G; FIBER: 2G; NET CARBS: 6G

FATHEAD BAGELS

PREP TIME: 20 MINUTES **COOK TIME:** 15 MINUTES

No need to miss bagels on your ketogenic diet! Use the FatHead base to create a variety of flavors of bagels from blueberry to cinnamon to pepperoni. This version keeps it simple with Everything Bagel Seasoning (page 247) on top. If you don't have a donut pan, you can place your round "wreaths" of dough onto a baking sheet lined with parchment paper or a silicone baking mat. *Serves 6*

¾ cup shredded mozzarella cheese

2 tablespoons cream cheese

¾ cup almond flour, plus additional as needed

1 large egg

Salt

Nonstick cooking spray

1 tablespoon Everything Bagel Seasoning (page 247)

1. Preheat the oven to 400°F.

2. In a microwave-safe bowl, add the mozzarella and cream cheese, and microwave on high for 1 minute. Stir the mixture and microwave again for 30 more seconds, until melted.

3. Add the almond flour and egg, and season with salt. Mix everything together gently.

4. If the dough is sticky, sprinkle it with a little extra almond flour. Wrap the dough in plastic wrap and place it in the refrigerator for 10 minutes to firm up.

5. Divide the dough into 6 balls and roll each out into a log.

6. Spray a donut pan with cooking spray and wrap the dough around the tin's indentations. Top with the everything bagel seasoning.

7. Bake the bagels for 15 minutes, until golden brown. Store leftovers in an airtight bag or container in the refrigerator for a week.

Variation: For a spicy alternative, you can top the dough with pepperoni and thin jalapeño pepper slices instead of everything bagel seasoning. Slice the bagels, toast, and top with cream cheese.

MACRONUTRIENTS	71% FAT	24% PROTEIN	5% CARBS

CALORIES: 88; TOTAL FAT: 7G; PROTEIN: 5G; TOTAL CARBS: 1G; FIBER: 0G; NET CARBS: 1G

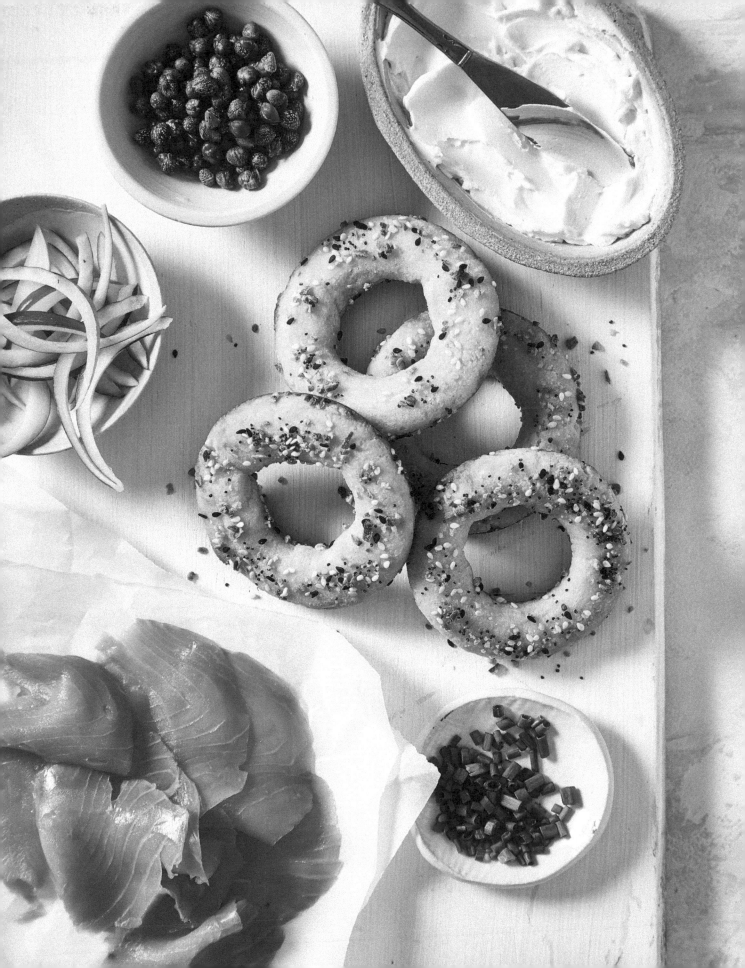

FATHEAD SAUSAGE BREAKFAST BISCUITS

PREP TIME: 10 MINUTES **COOK TIME:** 15 MINUTES

FatHead dough can be used in many different ways and allows you to get creative and create dishes inspired by high-carb favorites. In this book, we use it to create bagels, pizza, cinnamon rolls, and these delicious sausage-filled biscuits. *Serves 8*

○ COMFORT FOOD
○ SUPER QUICK

¾ cup shredded mozzarella cheese

2 tablespoons cream cheese

¾ cup almond flour, plus additional as needed

1 large egg

Salt

8 Sausage Patties (page 33)

¼ cup shredded Colby jack cheese

Nonstick cooking spray

1. Preheat the oven to 400°F.

2. In a microwave-safe bowl, combine the mozzarella and cream cheese, and microwave on high for 1 minute. Stir the mixture and microwave again for 30 more seconds, until melted.

3. Add the almond flour and egg, and season with salt. Mix everything together gently.

4. If the dough is sticky, sprinkle it with a little extra almond flour. Wrap the dough in plastic wrap and place it in the refrigerator for 10 minutes to firm up.

5. Divide the dough into 8 balls.

6. Spray a muffin tin with cooking spray and place the dough balls into the muffin cups.

7. Add a precooked sausage patty and Colby jack cheese on top of the dough in each cup and wrap the dough around both. Top each biscuit with a pinch more cheese.

8. Bake the breakfast biscuits for 15 minutes, until golden brown. Store leftovers in an airtight bag or container for a week in the refrigerator.

Variation: You can replace the sausage with leftover bacon and also add veggies if you wish.

MACRONUTRIENTS	69% FAT	29% PROTEIN	2% CARBS

CALORIES: 229; TOTAL FAT: 18G; PROTEIN: 16G; TOTAL CARBS: 1G; FIBER: 0G; NET CARBS: 1G

PORK RIND WAFFLES

PREP TIME: 5 MINUTES **COOK TIME:** 10 MINUTES

Pork rinds and waffles are a combination that is uniquely keto. Pork rinds can add flavor to all kinds of dishes, but in this one they give the waffle an amazing texture. Pour some keto-friendly syrup on top and enjoy your new favorite breakfast! *Serves 4*

○ COMFORT FOOD
● NUT-FREE
○ SUPER QUICK

4 large eggs

4 ounces cream cheese, at room temperature

1 teaspoon erythritol

2 teaspoons ground cinnamon

2 teaspoons vanilla extract

1½ teaspoons baking powder

4 tablespoons coconut flour

8 tablespoons ground pork rinds (ground in a food processor), divided

Nonstick cooking spray

1. Heat the waffle iron.

2. In the food processor, combine the eggs, cream cheese, erythritol, cinnamon, vanilla, baking powder, coconut flour, and 6 tablespoons of ground pork rinds. Thoroughly combine until you have a smooth consistency.

3. Spray the waffle iron with cooking spray and add ¼ to ½ cup of batter to it, depending on the size of your waffle iron. Sprinkle ½ tablespoon of ground pork rinds on top of each waffle, close, and cook until golden brown and crispy.

Variation: I also love to use these waffles as "bread" for a sandwich. A bacon grilled cheese with this pork rind–crusted waffle is heaven.

MACRONUTRIENTS	65% FAT	19% PROTEIN	16% CARBS

CALORIES: 248; TOTAL FAT: 17G; PROTEIN: 12G; TOTAL CARBS: 10G; FIBER: 6G; NET CARBS: 4G; ERYTHRITOL: 1G

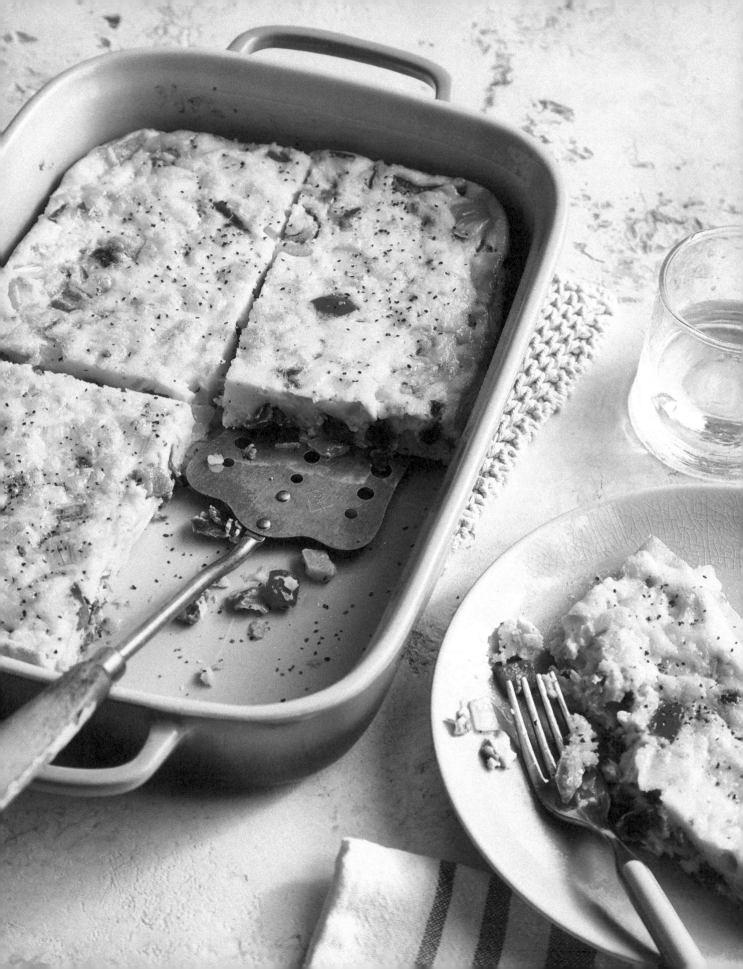

EGGS AND BREAKFAST

CHAPTER FIVE

Opposite: Denver Prosciutto Frittata

FETA, KALE, AND EGG BAKE WITH AVOCADO

PREP TIME: 10 MINUTES **COOK TIME:** 25 MINUTES

There's something extra fun about meals baked in individual ramekin dishes, and this recipe is no exception. This breakfast recipe can be customized in so many ways, but I especially love the flavor combination below served with a side of toasted keto-friendly bread. *Serves 2*

○ COMFORT FOOD
● NUT-FREE

Nonstick cooking spray

1 tablespoon extra-virgin olive oil

1 garlic clove, minced

1 shallot, sliced

2 cups chopped kale

¼ teaspoon red pepper flakes

2 large eggs

Salt

Freshly ground black pepper

¼ cup crumbled feta cheese

½ avocado, pitted, peeled, and cubed (optional)

1. Preheat the oven to 375°F.

2. Spray two ramekins with cooking spray.

3. In a skillet, heat the olive oil over medium heat and sauté the garlic and shallot for 2 to 3 minutes, until softened.

4. Add the kale and red pepper flakes to the skillet and cook for another 2 minutes.

5. Divide the kale between the ramekins and crack an egg into each. Season with salt and pepper.

6. Bake for 20 minutes, or until the egg whites are set.

7. Top with the feta cheese and avocado (if using) to serve.

Make It Paleo: Replace the feta with black olives to still get some good extra fat, but without the dairy.

MACRONUTRIENTS	65% FAT	19% PROTEIN	16% CARBS

CALORIES: 220; TOTAL FAT: 16G; PROTEIN: 11G; TOTAL CARBS: 9G; FIBER: 1G; NET CARBS: 8G

PARMESAN CLOUD EGGS

PREP TIME: 5 MINUTES **COOK TIME:** 8 MINUTES

The first time I saw cloud eggs I was amazed, and I couldn't believe I had never made these light, puffy creations before. Runny yolk in the middle of a flavorful cloud of egg whites and seasoning—yum! The key is getting the egg whites super fluffy, so use a mixer unless you are looking for an intense arm workout. *Serves 2*

○ COMFORT FOOD
● NUT-FREE
○ SUPER QUICK

4 large eggs, whites and yolks separated

Salt

2 cooked bacon slices, crumbled

1 scallion, finely chopped, green parts only

3 tablespoons grated Parmeson cheese

Freshly ground black pepper

1. Preheat the oven to 450°F.

2. Line a baking sheet with a silicone mat or parchment paper.

3. In a mixing bowl, combine the egg whites and salt (to taste). Using a mixer, beat on high until stiff.

4. Fold in the crumbled bacon, scallions, and Parmesan cheese.

5. Divide the egg white mixture into four mounds on the baking sheet. Create a nest in the middle of each mound—the egg yolk will go in there later.

6. Bake the mounds for about 3 minutes, until they're slightly golden.

7. Gently add a yolk to the middle of each nest. You can use a spoon to open up the nest a bit more if needed.

8. Bake for 3 to 5 minutes. You want the yolk to stay runny.

9. Remove the eggs and season with salt and pepper.

Make It Paleo: You can leave out the cheese, and they will still be delicious!

MACRONUTRIENTS	64% FAT	34% PROTEIN	2% CARBS

CALORIES: 187; TOTAL FAT: 13G; PROTEIN: 16G; TOTAL CARBS: 1G; FIBER: 0; NET CARBS: 1G

CAULIFLOWER EGG PUFFS

PREP TIME: 5 MINUTES **COOK TIME:** 25 MINUTES

The cauliflower in this recipe really changes the texture from a typical egg cup to something that has more of a muffin texture. This recipe is a great base, but feel free to get creative with other veggies or meats to add to the eggs and cauliflower. *Serves 6*

- DAIRY-FREE
- NUT-FREE
- PALEO OR PALEO-FRIENDLY
- SUPER QUICK

1 cup cauliflower florets

5 large eggs

1 cup chopped spinach

¾ cup cubed ham or pancetta

Salt

Freshly ground black pepper

Nonstick cooking spray

1. Preheat the oven to 350°F.

2. In a food processor, add the cauliflower and pulse several times until it is ground into rice-size pieces.

3. In a large bowl, whisk the eggs. Add the spinach, ham, and cauliflower rice. Season with salt and pepper and mix well.

4. Spray a muffin tin with cooking spray and divide the mixture into the muffin cups.

5. Bake for 25 minutes, until the eggs are set and golden.

Allergen Tip: You can use an egg replacement for this dish if you are allergic to eggs.

MACRONUTRIENTS	54% FAT	41% PROTEIN	5% CARBS

CALORIES: 96; TOTAL FAT: 6G; PROTEIN: 10G; TOTAL CARBS: 1G; FIBER: 1G; NET CARBS: 0G

PORTOBELLO BREAKFAST CUPS

PREP TIME: 5 MINUTES **COOK TIME:** 20 MINUTES

I love big, meaty portobello mushrooms, and they make a great vessel for dishes. These breakfast cups are rich and delicious. I adore having them for brunch, and they are easy to make for a crowd. Portobellos also make a great base for all kinds of ingredients, so get creative with cheese and meat toppings. *Serves 2*

● NUT-FREE
○ SUPER QUICK

2 large portobello mushrooms, stemmed

1 cup creamed spinach

2 large eggs

Salt

Freshly ground black pepper

¼ cup shredded Gruyère cheese

4 cooked bacon slices, crumbled

1. Preheat the oven to 375°F.

2. Place the mushrooms in a small baking dish, gill sides up.

3. Spoon the creamed spinach into the mushrooms. Create a well in the middle to make room for the egg.

4. Crack an egg into the middle of each mushroom, and season with salt and pepper. Add the cheese and bacon on top.

5. Bake for 20 minutes, until the eggs are set and the cheese is golden.

Variation: You can use 1 (10-ounce) package of frozen creamed spinach that is thawed if you wish.

MACRONUTRIENTS	60% FAT	29.5% PROTEIN	10.5% CARBS

CALORIES: 308; TOTAL FAT: 21G; PROTEIN: 23G; TOTAL CARBS: 10G; FIBER: 2G; NET CARBS: 8G

CHEESE SHELL BREAKFAST TACOS

PREP TIME: 10 MINUTES **COOK TIME:** 15 MINUTES

Miss the crunch of crispy taco shells? Cheese taco shells to the rescue! Cheese chips are one of my favorite snacks, so one day I decided to make slightly larger cheese chips and then bend them into taco shells while they were still pliable and ta-da! Pro tip: You can also make little bowls with them using muffin cups. There are just so many fun options with these. *Serves 2*

○ COMFORT FOOD
● NUT-FREE
○ SUPER QUICK

1⅓ cups shredded Mexican blend cheese

1 tablespoon butter or ghee

4 large eggs

2 tablespoons heavy whipping cream

Salt

Freshly ground black pepper

Dash hot sauce

1 avocado, pitted, peeled, and sliced or cubed

1 tablespoon chopped cilantro

1. Preheat the oven to 350°F. Line a baking sheet with a silicone baking mat or parchment paper.

2. Add ⅓-cup mounds of shredded cheese to the pan, leaving plenty of space between them. Bake until the edges are brown and the middle of each has fully melted, about 7 minutes.

3. Set the pan on the cooking rack. You will need to move quickly to bend the shells while they are still pliable. You can get creative with what you want to bend them over. I like to create a "rack" over my sink with a wider cooling rack to drape them over or sometimes over the sides of a larger storage container. As they cool, they will harden.

4. In a skillet, heat the butter over medium heat.

5. Whisk in the eggs and heavy cream, and season with salt, pepper, and a dash of hot sauce.

6. Scramble the eggs for 3 minutes, or to desired doneness.

7. Fill the cheese shells with the scrambled eggs, and top with the avocado and cilantro.

Variation: I love to use leftovers in tacos. Rotisserie chicken, crumbled bacon, or whatever else you have on hand would be a great addition.

MACRONUTRIENTS	75% FAT	21% PROTEIN	4% CARBS

CALORIES: 661; TOTAL FAT: 57G; PROTEIN: 33G; TOTAL CARBS: 8G; FIBER: 5G; NET CARBS: 3G

SMOKED SALMON EGGS BENEDICT

PREP TIME: 15 MINUTES **COOK TIME:** 5 MINUTES

I shied away from making this dish for so long because I have always been scared to poach eggs. I finally got over that and discovered it isn't so difficult after all. I replace the "bread" element of eggs Benedict with smoked salmon, and it's delicious. *Serves 2*

○ COMFORT FOOD
◐ DAIRY-FREE
● NUT-FREE
● PALEO OR PALEO-FRIENDLY
○ SUPER QUICK

1 teaspoon white vinegar

2 large eggs

8 ounces smoked salmon

¼ cup Dairy-Free Hollandaise Sauce (page 256)

1 tablespoon chopped fresh chives

1. Fill a saucepan half full with water and add the vinegar. Bring to a boil on high heat.

2. In two small bowls, carefully crack the eggs, keeping the yolks intact.

3. Once the water is boiling, lower the heat to medium and wait until it simmers.

4. Using a spoon, swirl the water so it looks like a whirlpool.

5. Very, very gently slide an egg into the water, and then the other.

6. Cook for 3 minutes for soft, 4 minutes for slightly set, and 5 minutes for set eggs. If desired, you can skim off any excess egg whites while they cook. When the eggs are cooked to your desired doneness, carefully remove them with a large spoon.

7. On two plates, divide the smoked salmon, top with the poached eggs, drizzle the hollandaise on top, and top with the chives.

Variation: If you are not dairy-free, add a Cloud Oopsie Roll (page 42) as a base.

MACRONUTRIENTS	64% FAT	36% PROTEIN	0% CARBS

CALORIES: 323; TOTAL FAT: 23G; PROTEIN: 29G; TOTAL CARBS: 0G; FIBER: 0G; NET CARBS: 0G

CHEESY SPINACH EGG BAKE
WITH PORK RIND DUST

PREP TIME: 10 MINUTES **COOK TIME:** 25 MINUTES

Pork rind dust is a magical thing that can be used anywhere you would normally use bread crumbs. You can buy preground pork rinds, but I just throw some of them in the food processor. There are a lot of flavors of pork rinds available these days, offering a great opportunity for experimentation. *Serves 2*

○ COMFORT FOOD

● NUT-FREE

Nonstick cooking spray

3 ounces fresh spinach

½ cup shredded Gruyère cheese, divided

4 large eggs

Salt

Freshly ground black pepper

1 tablespoon heavy whipping cream

¼ cup ground pork rinds

1 tablespoon chopped fresh parsley

1. Preheat the oven to 400°F.

2. Spray a 9-by-9-inch baking dish with cooking spray.

3. Place the spinach in the baking dish first, and top with ¼ cup of Gruyère cheese. Create four wells for the eggs.

4. Crack the eggs, one at a time, in a small bowl and then gently add one to each well.

5. Season the eggs with salt and pepper.

6. Drizzle the heavy cream over the baking dish and then add the remaining ¼ cup of Gruyère cheese. Sprinkle the ground pork rind dust over the spinach and cheese.

7. Bake for 25 minutes, or until the eggs reach your desired level of doneness. Garnish with the parsley.

Variation: You can also toss 2 diced Roma tomatoes into this dish. If you do, add the tomatoes to the baking dish first, then season and add the spinach.

MACRONUTRIENTS	67% FAT	29% PROTEIN	4% CARBS

CALORIES: 338; TOTAL FAT: 26G; PROTEIN: 25G; TOTAL CARBS: 3G; FIBER: 1G; NET CARBS: 2G

BREAKFAST BACON EGG SALAD CUPS

PREP TIME: 15 MINUTES **COOK TIME:** 15 MINUTES

I'm a huge fan of egg salad and really anything that involves eggs. I am also not one to confine a dish like egg salad to being just for lunch. I love the smooth texture of the egg salad paired with the crunch of crispy bacon and fresh lettuce. *Serves 2*

○ COMFORT FOOD

● NUT-FREE

○ SUPER QUICK

4 large eggs

2 tablespoons avocado oil mayonnaise

1 tablespoon sour cream

1 teaspoon Dijon mustard

1 tablespoon chopped chives or scallions

Salt

Freshly ground black pepper

4 romaine lettuce leaves

⅛ teaspoon paprika

4 bacon slices, cooked

1. In a medium saucepan, cover the eggs with water. Place the pan over high heat and bring the water to a boil. Once it is boiling, turn off the heat, cover, and leave on the burner for 10 to 12 minutes.

2. Remove the eggs with a slotted spoon and run them under cold water for 1 minute or submerge them in an ice bath. Gently tap the shells and peel. Run cold water over your hands as you remove the shells.

3. In a medium bowl, mash the eggs with a fork.

4. Add the mayonnaise, sour cream, and Dijon, and thoroughly mix until smooth. Add in the chives and season with salt and pepper.

5. Divide the egg salad into the romaine leaves. Sprinkle the paprika on top. Add 1 bacon slice to each cup, either whole or crumbled on top.

Make It Paleo: You can replace the mayonnaise and sour cream with one avocado.

MACRONUTRIENTS	68% FAT	26% PROTEIN	6% CARBS

CALORIES: 302; TOTAL FAT: 23G; PROTEIN: 19G; TOTAL CARBS: 5G; FIBER: 0G; NET CARBS: 5G

MEXICAN BREAKFAST BOWL

PREP TIME: 10 MINUTES **COOK TIME:** 20 MINUTES

I love any kind of pork for breakfast, and that includes carnitas. This is a super-filling dish that's also calorie dense, so I like to eat this as the larger of the two meals I eat daily. If Chipotle served breakfast, I imagine it would be something like this dish! *Serves 2*

○ COMFORT FOOD

● NUT-FREE

○ SUPER QUICK

1 tablespoon butter or ghee

1 cup Spicy Slow Cooker Shredded Pork (page 164)

4 large eggs

2 tablespoons heavy whipping cream

Salt

Freshly ground black pepper

½ cup shredded Mexican blend cheese

1 avocado, pitted, peeled, and sliced

¼ cup sour cream

1 tablespoon chopped cilantro

1 recipe Cauliflower Rice (page 36) (optional)

1. In a skillet, heat the butter over medium-high heat.

2. Add the pork and cook.

3. Meanwhile, in a small bowl, whisk the eggs and heavy cream, and season with salt and pepper.

4. When the pork is crisp on the edges, remove it from the skillet and divide it between two bowls. I like to push it to one half of the bowl, leaving room for the scrambled eggs.

5. Reduce the heat to medium, and scramble the eggs for 3 minutes, or to desired doneness.

6. Divide the eggs between the two bowls. Add the cheese, then the avocado slices, sour cream, and cilantro.

Variation: You can add cauliflower rice to this bowl to make it even more filling.

MACRONUTRIENTS	68% FAT	29% PROTEIN	3% CARBS

CALORIES: 680; TOTAL FAT: 50.5G; PROTEIN: 48.5G; TOTAL CARBS: 9G; FIBER: 4.5G; NET CARBS: 4.5G

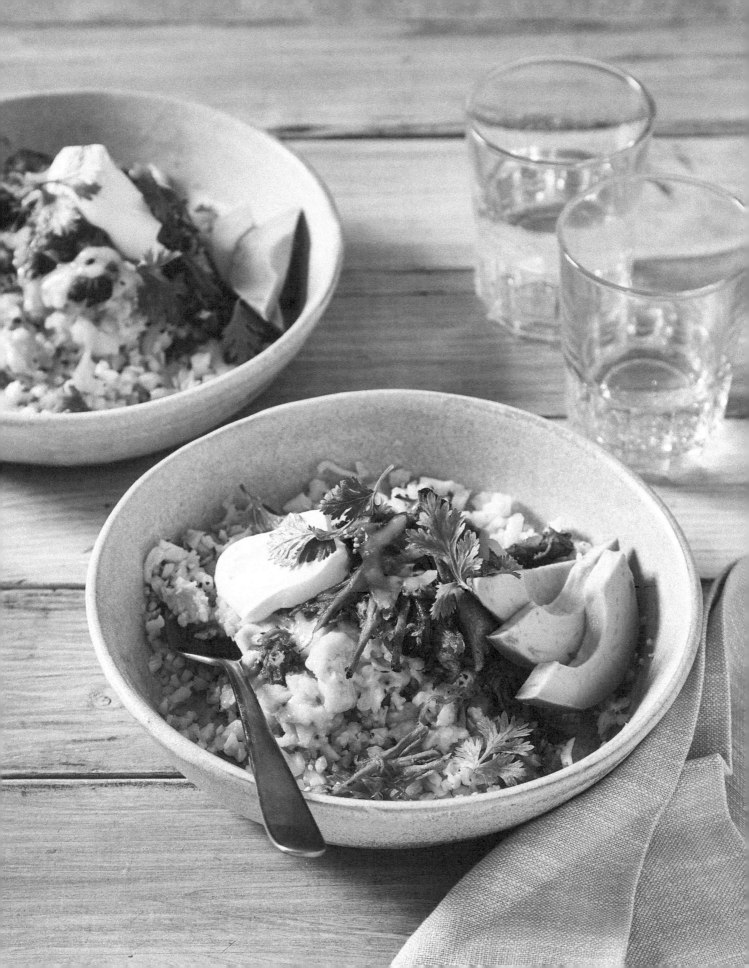

BREAKFAST NACHOS

PREP TIME: 5 MINUTES **COOK TIME:** 25 MINUTES

I love anything in nacho form. Pile on all the goodness! I love how every bite is different. These nachos are made of roasted cauliflower instead of carb-filled chips. Sound weird? They are amazing! *Serves 2*

○ COMFORT FOOD
◐ DAIRY-FREE
● NUT-FREE
● PALEO OR PALEO-FRIENDLY
○ SUPER QUICK

1½ cups cauliflower florets

2 tablespoons extra-virgin olive oil

¼ teaspoon ground cumin

¼ teaspoon paprika

¼ teaspoon chili powder

Salt

Freshly ground black pepper

2 large eggs

1 teaspoon white vinegar

½ cup Dairy-Free Avocado Crema (page 257)

½ cup Pico de Gallo (page 250)

¼ cup sliced jalapeño peppers

4 cooked bacon slices, crumbled

1. Preheat the oven to 425°F.

2. In a large bowl, toss the cauliflower florets, olive oil, cumin, paprika, and chili powder. Season with salt and pepper. Mix until the florets are evenly coated.

3. Spread the cauliflower on a baking sheet and roast for 25 minutes, until toasted and golden.

4. While the cauliflower is roasting, poach the eggs. Fill a saucepan half full with water and add the vinegar. Bring to a boil on high heat.

5. Crack the eggs into individual small bowls.

6. Once the water is boiling, lower the heat to medium and wait until it simmers.

7. Using a spoon, swirl the water so it looks like a whirlpool. Very, very gently slide one egg into the water and then the other. Cook for 3 minutes for soft, 4 minutes for slightly set, and 5 minutes for set. You can skim off any excess egg whites while they cook. When the eggs are cooked to your desired doneness, carefully remove them with a large spoon.

8. Divide the cauliflower between two bowls. Top each with the avocado crema, pico de gallo, and jalapeño slices. Add the poached eggs and crumbled bacon on top.

Allergen Tip: Although I love the runny egg on top, you can leave it off and the dish will be just as delicious!

| MACRONUTRIENTS | 77% FAT | 15% PROTEIN | 8% CARBS |

CALORIES: 407; TOTAL FAT: 35G; PROTEIN: 15G; TOTAL CARBS: 8G; FIBER: 4G; NET CARBS: 4G

BAKED CHORIZO EGGS

PREP TIME: 10 MINUTES **COOK TIME:** 30 MINUTES

I love this dish for breakfast or brunch, but it is wonderful any time of day. I don't buy chorizo very often, and whenever I make this, I wonder why I don't buy it more. It has such a great kick of spice! *Serves 2*

○ COMFORT FOOD
◑ DAIRY-FREE
● NUT-FREE
● PALEO

1 tablespoon avocado oil, coconut oil, or ghee

1 shallot, diced

1 garlic clove, minced

½ cup diced chorizo sausage

½ (14.5-ounce) can diced fire-roasted tomatoes

1 teaspoon chili powder

Dash hot sauce (optional)

1 cup chopped kale

4 large eggs

Salt

Freshly ground black pepper

2 tablespoons chopped fresh parsley

1. Preheat the oven to 400°F.

2. Heat a cast iron skillet over medium heat. Add the avocado oil, followed by the shallot, and cook while stirring for 1 to 2 minutes. Add the garlic and chorizo, and cook for 3 minutes, until the chorizo begins to brown.

3. Add the diced tomatoes, chili powder, and a dash of hot sauce (if using). Simmer the mixture for 6 minutes and then add the kale and cook until the kale is wilted, about 2 more minutes.

4. Create four wells in the mixture for the eggs. Crack an egg carefully into each well. Season the eggs with salt and pepper.

5. Place the skillet into the oven to cook the eggs for 12 minutes, or until the eggs are set to your liking.

6. Remove from the oven and garnish with the parsley.

Variation: If you prefer spinach, you can use it instead of kale.

MACRONUTRIENTS	66% FAT	23% PROTEIN	11% CARBS

CALORIES: 321; TOTAL FAT: 24G; PROTEIN: 19G; TOTAL CARBS: 10G; FIBER: 2G; NET CARBS: 8G

SAUSAGE AND EGG BREAKFAST JARS

PREP TIME: 10 MINUTES **COOK TIME:** 30 MINUTES

Mason jars are great for so many things, including baking beautiful egg dishes. Fluffy and flavorful, these eggs can be customized for each family member very easily. I also love how the jars look with the ingredients layered inside. *Serves 4*

○ COMFORT FOOD
● NUT-FREE
● PALEO

4 large eggs

4 egg whites

½ cup sour cream or Dairy-Free Sour Cream (page 259)

1 teaspoon garlic powder

¼ teaspoon red pepper flakes

2 tablespoons butter or ghee, for greasing

2 cooked sausage links, diced

1 cup spinach

Salt

Freshly ground black pepper

1. Preheat the oven to 350°F.

2. In a large mixing bowl, combine the eggs, egg whites, sour cream, garlic powder, and red pepper flakes. Using a mixer beat until fluffy.

3. Grease four pint-size mason jars with butter or ghee.

4. Divide the sausage and spinach between the jars. Pour in the egg mixture until the jars are three-quarters full. The mixture will rise as it bakes.

5. Place the jars on a baking sheet and bake for 25 to 30 minutes. Remove when the eggs are firm.

6. Cool the jars for 10 minutes and season with salt and pepper.

Variation: Breakfast jars can be customized with all kinds of ingredients, and this is the perfect opportunity to use leftover veggies or greens.

MACRONUTRIENTS	60% FAT	35% PROTEIN	5% CARBS

CALORIES: 254; TOTAL FAT: 22G; PROTEIN: 13G; TOTAL CARBS: 3G; FIBER: 1G; NET CARBS: 2G

SANTA FE EGG MUFFINS

PREP TIME: 5 MINUTES **COOK TIME:** 25 MINUTES

Egg muffins are great for making ahead of time and then heating up when you need a quick breakfast. These ones are filled with ingredients that remind me of when I lived in Santa Fe. I use precooked chorizo sausage in this recipe to keep it quick and easy. *Serves 6*

○ COMFORT FOOD
● NUT-FREE
○ SUPER QUICK

5 large eggs

¼ cup heavy whipping cream

Salt

Freshly ground black pepper

Nonstick cooking spray

½ cup diced red bell peppers

½ cup diced chorizo sausage

2 ounces canned green chiles, drained

1 chopped scallion, green parts only

¼ cup shredded pepper jack cheese

1. Preheat the oven to 350°F.

2. In a large bowl, whisk the eggs and heavy cream. Season with salt and pepper.

3. Spray a muffin tin with cooking spray.

4. Divide the bell peppers, chorizo, green chiles, and scallions between the muffin cups. Pour the egg mixture over the vegetables.

5. Divide the cheese on top of each muffin cup.

6. Bake for 25 minutes, until set.

Make It Paleo: You can leave out the cheese or replace it with a dairy-free option. You can also replace the heavy whipping cream with full-fat coconut milk.

MACRONUTRIENTS	72% FAT	23% PROTEIN	5% CARBS

CALORIES: 172; TOTAL FAT: 14G; PROTEIN: 10G; TOTAL CARBS: 2G; FIBER: 1G; NET CARBS: 1G

DENVER PROSCIUTTO FRITTATA

PREP TIME: 5 MINUTES **COOK TIME:** 30 MINUTES

Frittatas are one of my all-time favorite breakfasts. Making these is so much faster than making omelets since you can mix everything together and then throw it all in the oven. I don't add cheese to my frittatas because I find them fluffier without, but you can if you wish. I'm calling this one a "Denver" frittata, but replacing the usual ham with prosciutto. *Serves 4*

○ COMFORT FOOD

● NUT-FREE

2 tablespoons butter or ghee, divided

¼ cup chopped green, red, or yellow bell pepper

½ onion, chopped

4 ounces prosciutto, chopped

8 large eggs

1 cup heavy whipping cream

Salt

Freshly ground black pepper

1. Preheat the oven to 375°F. Coat a 9-by-12-inch baking pan with 1 tablespoon of butter.

2. In a small skillet, melt the remaining 1 tablespoon of butter over medium-high heat. Add the pepper and onion, and cook for about 4 minutes, until softened. Remove the skillet from the heat, add the prosciutto, and mix well.

3. Transfer the mixture to the baking pan.

4. In a large bowl, whisk the eggs and cream. Season with salt and pepper. Pour the mixture over the vegetable-prosciutto mixture.

5. Bake for 25 minutes, or until the edges are golden and the eggs are just set.

6. Cool for 5 minutes and then cut into 4 portions.

Make Ahead: I love making this frittata on the weekend and then saving a couple of pieces to reheat. It takes only about 30 seconds in the microwave.

MACRONUTRIENTS	78% FAT	19% PROTEIN	3% CARBS

CALORIES: 473; TOTAL FAT: 41G; PROTEIN: 22G; TOTAL CARBS: 4G; FIBER: 0G; NET CARBS: 4G

BACON SRIRACHA DEVILED EGGS

PREP TIME: 30 MINUTES

Spice up your morning (or any time of day) with this fun take on deviled eggs. The spicy Sriracha, which is made with red chiles, adds a nice kick, especially in combination with the salty crisp of the bacon on top. *Serves 6*

○ COMFORT FOOD
● NUT-FREE
○ SUPER QUICK

6 large eggs, hard-boiled

¼ cup avocado oil mayonnaise

2 tablespoons sour cream

1½ tablespoons Sriracha

½ teaspoon paprika

3 bacon slices, cooked and chopped

1. Halve the eggs lengthwise. With a small spoon, carefully remove the yolks, transfer them to a small bowl, and mash them.

2. Add the mayonnaise, sour cream, and Sriracha, and mix with a fork until smooth.

3. Spoon or pipe the yolk mixture back into the egg whites. I put the yolk mixture in a small plastic ziptop bag, cut off the corner, and pipe it in that way.

4. Top each egg with paprika and a bite-size piece of crispy bacon.

Make Ahead: The eggs store well in an airtight container, but the bacon will get soggy if it's on top, so store that separately.

MACRONUTRIENTS	69% FAT	23% PROTEIN	8% CARBS

CALORIES: 70; TOTAL FAT: 5G; PROTEIN: 4G; TOTAL CARBS: 2G; FIBER: 0G; NET CARBS: 2G

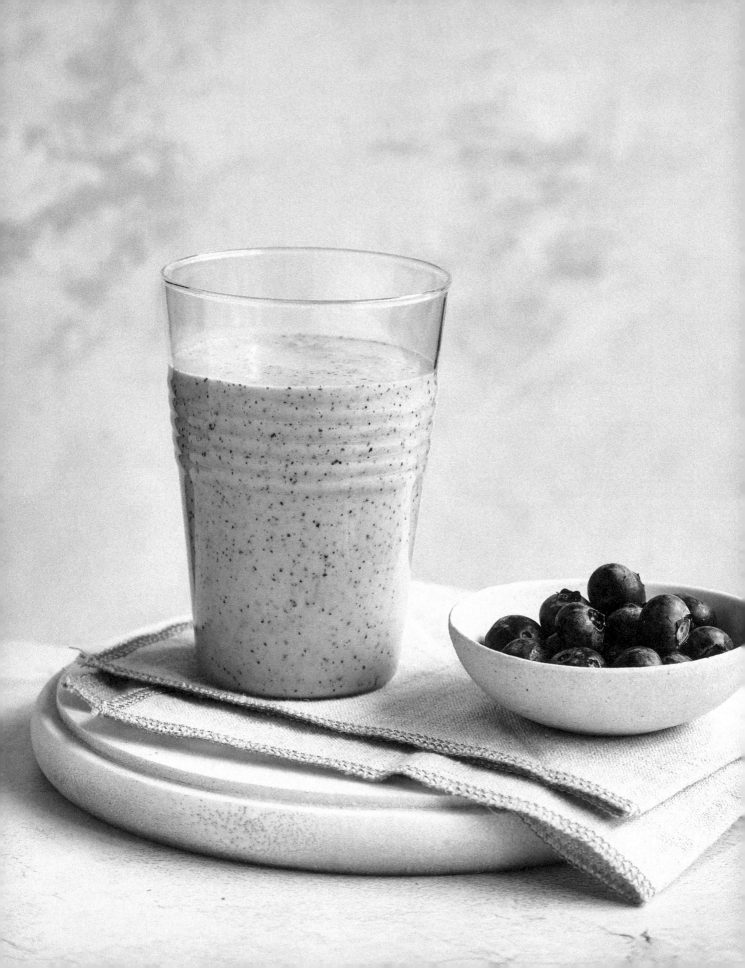

BEVERAGES AND SMOOTHIES

CHAPTER SIX

Opposite: Blueberry-Coconut Smoothie

FATTY LATTE

PREP TIME: 5 MINUTES **COOK TIME:** 5 MINUTES

In my first book I shared the most basic recipe for Bulletproof coffee, but the fun part about "fatty coffees" is that there are so many different ways to make them. This one is dairy-free. I love adding the cinnamon and vanilla extract, but you can also add other flavorings if you wish. The collagen is completely optional, but it has so many healing properties. *Serves 1*

- DAIRY-FREE
- NUT-FREE
- PALEO OR PALEO-FRIENDLY
- SUPER QUICK

½ cup full-fat coconut milk

2 teaspoons MCT oil or Bulletproof Brain Octane Oil

1½ cups hot brewed coffee

1 tablespoon ghee

½ teaspoon ground cinnamon

¼ teaspoon vanilla extract

1 scoop collagen powder (optional)

1. In a saucepan, combine the coconut milk and MCT oil, and heat over medium heat.

2. In a blender, combine the hot coffee, hot coconut milk mixture, ghee, cinnamon, and vanilla. Blend on high for 15 to 30 seconds, until frothy.

3. Add the collagen (if using) and process on the lowest setting until fully combined. Collagen molecules are delicate and can be harmed on high blending.

Variation: There are great grass-fed collagen products available in a variety of flavors that can add great flavor to your coffee. The collagen powder adds protein, so if you are looking to avoid protein in the morning, leave it out.

MACRONUTRIENTS (WITHOUT COLLAGEN)	94% FAT	2% PROTEIN	4% CARBS

CALORIES: 423; TOTAL FAT: 47G; PROTEIN: 2G; TOTAL CARBS: 4G; FIBER: 1G; NET CARBS: 3G

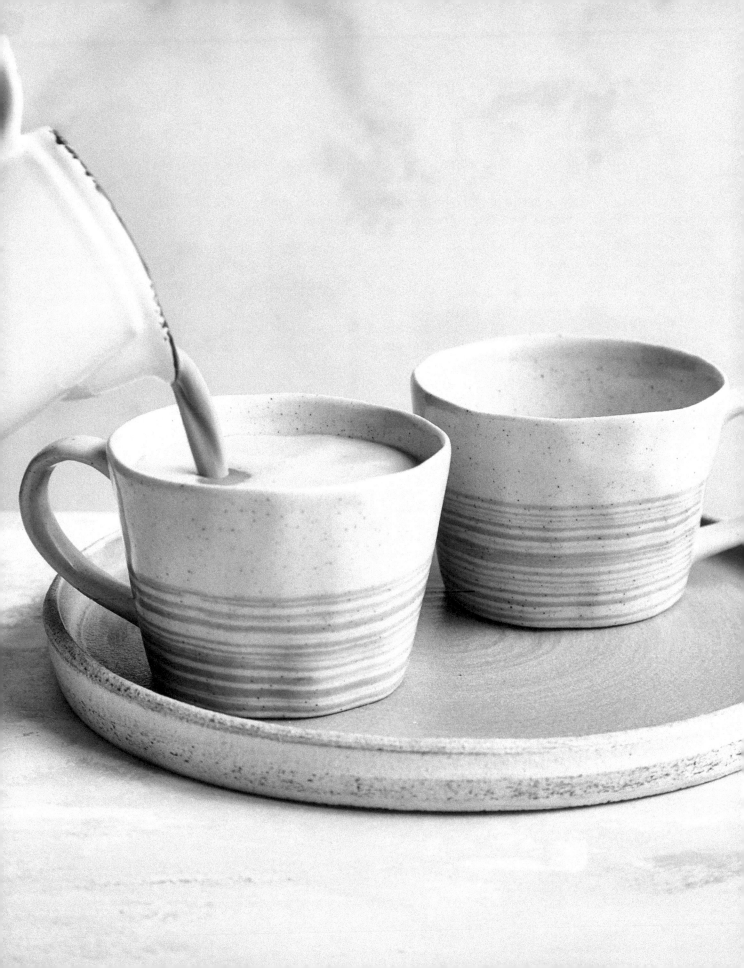

FATTY ICED COFFEE

PREP TIME: 5 MINUTES

Anyone who has tried to ice regular Bulletproof coffee, with butter or coconut oil, knows that you end up with a bunch of frozen chunks in your drink, which is not appetizing at all. This version uses full-fat coconut milk and MCT oil, so it is frothy, dairy-free, and delicious. *Serves 1*

- ● ALLERGEN-FREE
- ○ COMFORT FOOD
- ◐ DAIRY-FREE
- ● NUT-FREE
- ● PALEO OR PALEO-FRIENDLY
- ○ SUPER QUICK

1½ cups brewed coffee, chilled

¼ cup full-fat coconut milk

2 teaspoons MCT oil or Bulletproof Brain Octane Oil

1 cup ice

¼ teaspoon vanilla extract

1 scoop collagen powder (optional)

1. In a blender, add the coffee, coconut milk, MCT oil, ice, and vanilla, and blend on high for 15 to 30 seconds, until frothy.

2. Add the collagen (if using) and process on the lowest setting until fully combined. Collagen molecules are delicate and can be harmed on high blending.

Make Ahead: This may seem obvious, but it's tried and true: Chill your coffee in the refrigerator overnight so it is ready to go in the morning.

MACRONUTRIENTS	95% FAT	3% PROTEIN	2% CARBS

CALORIES: 189; TOTAL FAT: 21G; PROTEIN: 1G; TOTAL CARBS: 2G; FIBER: 0G; NET CARBS: 2G

FATTY TEA

PREP TIME: 5 MINUTES

If you are looking for a way to get fats into a warm beverage but aren't in the mood for coffee, then fatty tea is perfect for you. You can use any tea you wish, but I like to use chai. *Serves 1*

- ● ALLERGEN-FREE
- ○ DAIRY-FREE
- ● NUT-FREE
- ● PALEO OR PALEO-FRIENDLY
- ○ SUPER QUICK

1½ cups hot brewed tea

1 tablespoon full-fat coconut milk

2 teaspoons MCT oil or Bulletproof Brain Octane Oil

1 scoop collagen powder (optional)

½ teaspoon ground cinnamon

1. In a blender, combine the tea, coconut milk, and MCT oil. Blend on high for 15 to 30 seconds, until frothy.

2. Add the collagen (if using) and mix on low until combined.

3. Pour the tea into a mug and sprinkle the cinnamon on top.

Variation: You can also add ingredients with health benefits like turmeric into your tea mixture.

MACRONUTRIENTS	69% FAT	28% PROTEIN	3% CARBS

CALORIES: 155; TOTAL FAT: 12G; PROTEIN: 11G; TOTAL CARBS: 1G; FIBER: 1G; NET CARBS: 0G

FATTY MATCHA

PREP TIME: 5 MINUTES

Matcha is super hot right now, and for good reason: It is really high in antioxidants. It also tastes great, and when combined with some healthy fats, it makes an incredible alternative to fatty coffee. *Serves 1*

⬤ ALLERGEN-FREE
◯ DAIRY-FREE
⬤ NUT-FREE
⬤ PALEO OR PALEO-FRIENDLY
◯ SUPER QUICK

1 teaspoon matcha powder

½ cup boiling water

¼ cup full-fat coconut milk

1 teaspoon MCT oil or Bulletproof Brain Octane Oil

Erythritol (optional)

½ teaspoon ground cinnamon

1. In a small bowl, combine the matcha and boiling water, and whisk until combined. If you have a frother, you can use it instead.

2. In a blender, combine the matcha mixture, coconut milk, MCT oil, and erythritol (if using). Blend for 15 to 30 seconds.

3. Sprinkle the cinnamon on the top.

Variation: To make this even easier, there are matcha powders available that include powdered MCT oil in them.

MACRONUTRIENTS	90% FAT	4% PROTEIN	6% CARBS

CALORIES: 163; TOTAL FAT: 17G; PROTEIN: 2G; TOTAL CARBS: 3G; FIBER: 1G; NET CARBS: 2G

PINK PASSION ICED TEA

PREP TIME: 5 MINUTES

This will satisfy your desire for a glass of cold, refreshing iced tea, but it also has the benefit of additional healthy fat from the coconut milk. You can replace the vanilla extract and optional erythritol with a sugar-free coffee syrup if you wish. *Serves 1*

- ALLERGEN-FREE
- DAIRY-FREE
- NUT-FREE
- PALEO OR PALEO-FRIENDLY
- SUPER QUICK

1½ cups hot brewed Tazo® Passion Herbal Tea, chilled

¼ cup full-fat coconut milk

Erythritol (optional)

¼ teaspoon vanilla extract

1 cup ice

In a tall glass, combine the tea, coconut milk, erythritol (if using), and vanilla and stir. Add the ice.

Variation: You can try this with a variety of other herbal teas. I prefer fruity varieties, but feel free to experiment.

MACRONUTRIENTS	90% FAT	3% PROTEIN	7% CARBS

CALORIES: 114; TOTAL FAT: 12G; PROTEIN: 1G; TOTAL CARBS: 2G; FIBER: 0G; NET CARBS: 2G

FATTY HOT CHOCOLATE

PREP TIME: 5 MINUTES **COOK TIME:** 5 MINUTES

Hot chocolate is an essential comfort food for me. This version is dairy-free and super easy to make! *Serves 1*

- ● ALLERGEN-FREE
- ○ COMFORT FOOD
- ◐ DAIRY-FREE
- ● NUT-FREE
- ● PALEO OR PALEO-FRIENDLY
- ○ SUPER QUICK

1 cup full-fat coconut milk

1½ tablespoons cacao powder

¼ teaspoon ground cinnamon

1 tablespoon erythritol

¼ teaspoon vanilla extract or peppermint extract

Pinch salt

Dairy-Free Coconut Cream Whipped Cream (page 255)

1. In a small saucepan, heat the coconut milk over low heat, until it bubbles slightly.

2. While the coconut milk is heating, in a blender, combine the cacao, cinnamon, erythritol, vanilla, and a pinch salt. Add the warm coconut milk to the blender and process for 30 to 60 seconds, until fully mixed.

3. Top with the coconut cream whipped cream and serve.

MACRONUTRIENTS	90% FAT	4% PROTEIN	6% CARBS

CALORIES: 465; TOTAL FAT: 49G; PROTEIN: 6G; TOTAL CARBS: 14G; FIBER: 3G; NET CARBS: 11G; ERYTHRITOL: 12G

FATTY PUMPKIN SPICE LATTE

PREP TIME: 5 MINUTES **COOK TIME:** 10 MINUTES

Every year when fall rolls around, I find myself craving a PSL, so creating a keto-friendly version was a must! This will keep you full for hours and feeling cozy. Be sure to purchase pumpkin purée without added sugars (in other words, don't buy pumpkin pie mix), as that would defeat the purpose! *Serves 1*

- DAIRY-FREE
- ● NUT-FREE
- ● PALEO OR PALEO-FRIENDLY
- ○ SUPER QUICK

½ cup full-fat coconut milk

1 tablespoon butter or ghee

2 teaspoons MCT oil or Bulletproof Brain Octane Oil

1 to 2 tablespoons pumpkin purée

½ teaspoon pumpkin pie spice

¼ teaspoon vanilla extract

Erythritol (optional)

1½ cups hot brewed coffee

1. In a small saucepan, combine the coconut milk, butter, MCT oil, pumpkin purée, pumpkin pie spice, vanilla, and erythritol (if using). Bring to a simmer over medium heat for 5 to 7 minutes, stirring frequently.

2. In a blender, combine the saucepan mixture and the hot coffee.

3. Blend on high for 15 to 30 seconds, until frothy.

Variation: Turmeric is also a great addition to a pumpkin spice latte and provides anti-inflammatory benefits while aiding with digestion. Add just ¼ teaspoon of ground turmeric to the rest of the ingredients in the saucepan.

MACRONUTRIENTS	93% FAT	2% PROTEIN	5% CARBS

CALORIES: 409; TOTAL FAT: 45G; PROTEIN: 3G; TOTAL CARBS: 6G; FIBER: 1G; NET CARBS: 5G

FATTY COLD BREW NUT BUTTER LATTE

PREP TIME: 5 MINUTES

Cold brew coffee is everywhere now, so whether you make your own or pick one up at the store, this recipe takes it to another level. I'm calling this a latte, but for me it's really more like a rich, creamy dessert, even though it's appropriate for any time of day. *Serves 1*

○ DAIRY-FREE

● PALEO OR PALEO-FRIENDLY

○ SUPER QUICK

8 ounces cold brew coffee

½ cup full-fat coconut milk

1 tablespoon nut butter

2 teaspoons MCT oil or Bulletproof Brain Octane Oil

¼ teaspoon ground cinnamon

Pinch salt

Erythritol (optional)

1 tablespoon cacao nibs or powder

1. In a blender, combine the coffee, coconut milk, nut butter, MCT oil, cinnamon, salt, and erythritol (if using). If you are using cacao powder, add it now as well, but if you are using nibs, add them after blending. Blend for 30 seconds, until smooth and frothy.

2. Pour into a glass and sprinkle with the cacao nibs.

Variation: In all of the fatty coffee recipes I call for 2 teaspoons of MCT oil or Bulletproof Brain Octane Oil. This is a good "beginner" amount to ease into the ingredient because it can cause some stomach discomfort if you drink too much too fast. You can work your way up to 1 to 2 tablespoons as your body adjusts, which will add healthy fats (and calories).

MACRONUTRIENTS	88% FAT	5% PROTEIN	7% CARBS

CALORIES: 468; TOTAL FAT: 49G; PROTEIN: 7G; TOTAL CARBS: 12G; FIBER: 5G; NET CARBS: 7G

NUT BUTTER SMOOTHIE

PREP TIME: 5 MINUTES

I've become a big fan of nut butter in the last couple of years. Now I love to experiment with nut butters that have different nut combinations and unique flavors. *Serves 1*

○ COMFORT FOOD
◐ DAIRY-FREE
● PALEO OR PALEO-FRIENDLY
○ SUPER QUICK

1 tablespoon nut butter of your choice

½ cup full-fat coconut milk

½ teaspoon vanilla extract

1 cup ice

In a blender, combine the nut butter, coconut milk, vanilla, and ice, and blend for 30 to 60 seconds, until fully mixed.

Variation: Depending on the nut butter you choose, you may want to add erythritol to taste.

MACRONUTRIENTS	85% FAT	6% PROTEIN	9% CARBS

CALORIES: 330; TOTAL FAT: 34G; PROTEIN: 5G; TOTAL CARBS: 7G; FIBER: 1G; NET CARBS: 6G

BLUEBERRY-COCONUT SMOOTHIE

PREP TIME: 5 MINUTES

I love all things blueberry, so it is no surprise that I like this smoothie. It's a little different from most smoothies I make because there is no ice in it, which makes it super creamy. It's a little high in net carbs but can be as filling as a full meal and will leave you feeling satisfied. I like to drink this when I have a high-protein meal planned for later in the day. *Serves 1*

- ● ALLERGEN-FREE
- ◐ DAIRY-FREE
- ● NUT-FREE
- ● PALEO OR PALEO-FRIENDLY
- ○ SUPER QUICK

¼ cup blueberries

1 cup full-fat coconut milk

½ teaspoon vanilla extract

1 teaspoon MCT oil or Bulletproof Brain Octane Oil

Erythritol (optional)

In a blender, combine the blueberries, coconut milk, vanilla, MCT oil, and erythritol (if using). Blend until fully mixed, 30 to 60 seconds.

Variation: You can also swap out the blueberries for strawberries or blackberries. Add a scoop of collagen for added health benefits.

MACRONUTRIENTS	88% FAT	3% PROTEIN	9% CARBS

CALORIES: 506; TOTAL FAT: 53G; PROTEIN: 5G; TOTAL CARBS: 12G; FIBER: 1G; NET CARBS: 11G

MINT CACAO CHIP SMOOTHIE

PREP TIME: 5 MINUTES

Smoothies that feel like a dessert are my favorite because dessert time is usually when I crave them, and this mint cacao chip smoothie definitely fits the bill. This truly could be a dessert or a meal since it's relatively healthy but tastes decadent. The coconut cream whipped cream makes it feel extra special. *Serves 1*

○ DAIRY-FREE

● PALEO OR PALEO-FRIENDLY

○ SUPER QUICK

½ cup unsweetened almond milk

½ cup full-fat coconut milk

1 tablespoon cacao powder

½ avocado, pitted and peeled

¼ teaspoon mint extract or fresh mint leaves

1 teaspoon MCT oil or Bulletproof Brain Octane Oil

Erythritol (optional)

1 cup ice

½ tablespoon cacao nibs

Dairy-Free Coconut Cream Whipped Cream (page 255), for topping

1. In a blender, combine the almond milk, coconut milk, cacao powder, avocado, mint extract, MCT oil, erythritol (if using), and ice. Blend for 30 to 60 seconds, until fully combined.

2. Stir in the cacao nibs.

3. Top with coconut cream whipped cream.

Variation: As with any of these recipes, if you prefer another "milk" over coconut milk (such as heavy whipping cream, almond milk, or macadamia milk), feel free to substitute it in.

MACRONUTRIENTS	83% FAT	4% PROTEIN	13% CARBS

CALORIES: 415; TOTAL FAT: 41G; PROTEIN: 5G; TOTAL CARBS: 16G; FIBER: 7G; NET CARBS: 9G

AVOCADO TURMERIC SMOOTHIE

PREP TIME: 5 MINUTES

This green smoothie is full of vitamins. Avocados act very similar to bananas in smoothies, as they help thicken and hold everything together. Since I have autoimmune disorders, I love to incorporate turmeric whenever I can because of its anti-inflammatory properties. *Serves 1*

○ DAIRY-FREE
● PALEO OR PALEO-FRIENDLY
○ SUPER QUICK

½ avocado, pitted and peeled

¼ cup unsweetened almond milk

¼ cup full-fat coconut milk

½ teaspoon ground turmeric

1 teaspoon freshly squeezed lime juice

Erythritol (optional)

½ cup ice

In a blender, combine the avocado, almond milk, coconut milk, turmeric, lime juice, and erythritol (if using). Blend on high for 30 to 60 seconds. Add the ice and blend until smooth.

Variation: Add 1 teaspoon of chia seeds to the glass after blending. You can also add a handful of fresh spinach to the blender for even more vitamins.

MACRONUTRIENTS	81% FAT	4% PROTEIN	15% CARBS

CALORIES: 239; TOTAL FAT: 23G; PROTEIN: 3G; TOTAL CARBS: 9G; FIBER: 5G; NET CARBS: 4G

KETO-CHATA

PREP TIME: 5 MINUTES

Traditional horchata is so creamy, with a delicious combination of cinnamon and vanilla. This recipe may not be 100 percent authentic, but it is a yummy keto alternative to the sugar-filled version. Check out the boozy variation below; vodka has zero carbs, making a celebratory addition if you're so inclined! *Serves 1*

- ◐ DAIRY-FREE
- ● PALEO OR PALEO-FRIENDLY
- ○ SUPER QUICK

¼ cup unsweetened almond milk

¼ cup full-fat coconut milk

½ teaspoon ground cinnamon

¼ teaspoon vanilla extract

Erythritol (optional)

½ cup ice

1. In a blender, combine the almond milk, coconut milk, cinnamon, vanilla, and erythritol (if using). Blend on high for 30 seconds.

2. Add the ice and blend for 30 more seconds, until fully combined.

Variation: You can add some vodka to this combination and have a delicious keto version of a White Russian.

MACRONUTRIENTS	82% FAT	5% PROTEIN	13% CARBS

CALORIES: 131; TOTAL FAT: 13G; PROTEIN: 1G; TOTAL CARBS: 5G; FIBER: 1G; NET CARBS: 4G

KETO-JITO

PREP TIME: 5 MINUTES

I love a good mojito, and this keto version is delicious. Of course, cocktails don't have any nutritional value, but I still love having low-carb options when I'm in the mood for a drink (or two). *Serves 1*

● ALLERGEN-FREE
○ COMFORT FOOD
◐ DAIRY-FREE
● NUT-FREE
● PALEO OR PALEO-FRIENDLY
○ SUPER QUICK

¼ cup loosely packed fresh mint leaves

1 ounce freshly squeezed lime juice

1 teaspoon confectioners' erythritol

1 cup ice

2 ounces white rum

4 ounces club soda

1. In a tall glass, muddle the mint using the handle of a wooden spoon.

2. Add the lime juice and erythritol, and mix.

3. Add the ice and then pour in the rum and club soda. Stir again.

Variation: I also like to muddle blackberries into this for an extra-special keto-jito.

MACRONUTRIENTS	0% FAT	0% PROTEIN	100% CARBS

CALORIES: 130; TOTAL FAT: 0G; PROTEIN: 0G; TOTAL CARBS: 1G; FIBER: 0G; NET CARBS: 1G

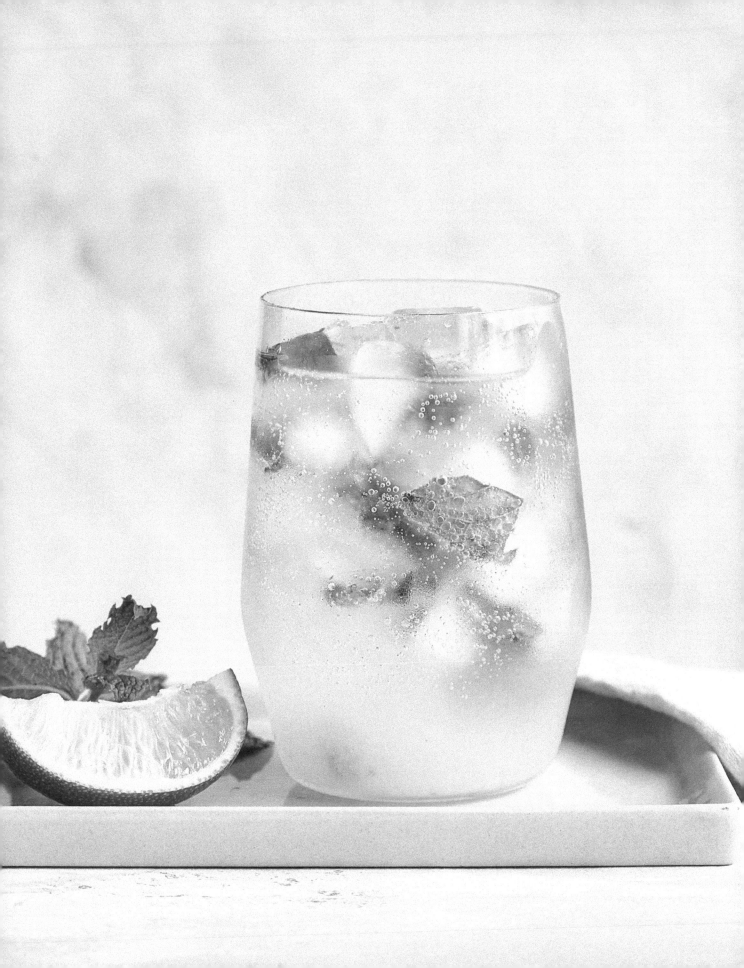

VODKA SODA

PREP TIME: 5 MINUTES

Personally, I enjoy low-carb cocktails, and this is my go-to drink when I'm out with friends. You will want to make sure you choose a gluten-free vodka, as many are not, but it is easy to find brands that are. If you are trying to lose weight, you will want to limit your alcohol consumption, as your body will have to burn the alcohol off before it can go back to burning fat. *Serves 1*

- ● ALLERGEN-FREE
- ○ COMFORT FOOD
- ◐ DAIRY-FREE
- ● NUT-FREE
- ● PALEO OR PALEO-FRIENDLY
- ○ SUPER QUICK

½ cup ice

2 ounces vodka

4 ounces club soda

1 lime wedge

In a glass, add the ice, pour in the vodka, and add the soda water. Garnish with the lime wedge. Voila!

Variation: I also like to add an ounce or two of other sugar-free naturally carbonated drinks for extra flavor. Be aware that tonic water is filled with sugar, and diet tonic is usually not available at bars and restaurants, so plain soda water is often your best option when you are out.

MACRONUTRIENTS	0% FAT	0% PROTEIN	100% CARBS

CALORIES: 128; TOTAL FAT: 0G; PROTEIN: 0G; TOTAL CARBS: 1G; FIBER: 0G; NET CARBS: 1G; ERYTHRITOL: 3G

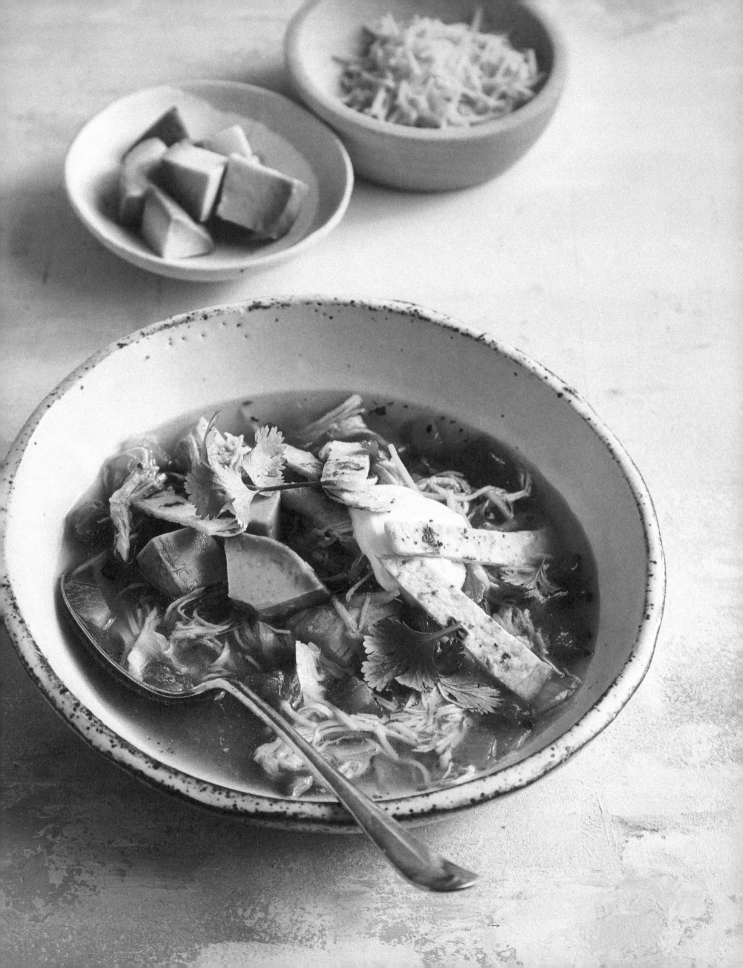

SOUPS AND SALADS

CHAPTER SEVEN

Opposite: Chicken Tortilla Soup

SPINACH AND ARTICHOKE "DIP" SOUP

PREP TIME: 5 MINUTES **COOK TIME:** 30 MINUTES

Spinach and artichoke dip has to be one of my favorite comfort foods, so I figured the rich flavors of the dip would also work really well in a soup! I make this with chicken bone broth, which has extra collagen, but you can use regular chicken broth, too. *Serves 4*

● NUT-FREE
○ COMFORT FOOD

2 tablespoons butter or ghee

½ onion, diced

2 garlic cloves, minced

4 ounces frozen spinach

¾ cup canned artichoke hearts, drained and chopped

2 cups chicken broth or chicken bone broth

½ cup heavy whipping cream

4 ounces cream cheese

½ cup grated Parmesan cheese, plus 1 tablespoon

Salt

Freshly ground black pepper

1. In a large pot, melt the butter over medium-high heat. Add the onion and sauté for about 3 minutes, until softened. Add the garlic and sauté for another 1 minute.

2. Add the spinach and, as it warms, break up any chunks. Cook for 5 minutes. Add the artichoke hearts and stir everything to combine.

3. Add the chicken broth and cook for 10 minutes.

4. Adjust the heat to low and add the heavy cream. Add the cream cheese, allowing it to melt and incorporate slowly for about 10 minutes. Stir occasionally, but do not turn the heat higher or the dairy will curdle.

5. Add ½ cup of Parmesan cheese and stir. Season with salt and pepper.

6. To serve, garnish the bowls with the remaining 1 tablespoon of Parmesan cheese.

Make Ahead: This soup reheats really well, which is why I always make enough for four people, even though there are only two of us in my household.

MACRONUTRIENTS	76% FAT	13% PROTEIN	11% CARBS

CALORIES: 395; TOTAL FAT: 34G; PROTEIN: 12G; TOTAL CARBS: 14G; FIBER: 2G; NET CARBS: 12G

CREAMY GREEN CHILE CHICKEN SOUP

PREP TIME: 5 MINUTES **COOK TIME:** 8 HOURS

I used to live in Santa Fe, where green chiles are worshipped and are incorporated into pretty much anything you can think of. This soup has a nice green chile kick and will fill your house with amazing smells as it cooks. If you are shy about spice, you can halve the amount of diced green chiles and then top this with cool cream cheese and avocado. *Serves 4*

○ COMFORT FOOD
● NUT-FREE

½ cup water

2 cups chicken broth or chicken bone broth

¾ cup salsa verde or green chile enchilada sauce

½ cup canned diced green chiles

1 tablespoon ground cumin

1 teaspoon garlic powder

1 teaspoon onion powder

2 to 3 boneless chicken breasts

Salt

Freshly ground black pepper

4 ounces cream cheese or Dairy-Free Cream Cheese (page 258), cubed

½ avocado, sliced, for serving

2 tablespoons sour cream or Dairy-Free Sour Cream (page 259), for serving

¼ cup shredded Mexican blend cheese, for serving

1. Turn the slow cooker to the low heat setting.

2. In the slow cooker, put the water, chicken broth, salsa verde, green chiles, cumin, garlic powder, and onion powder. Stir to combine.

3. Add the chicken breasts, cover, and cook for 7 hours.

4. When the cooking is complete, remove the chicken breasts, shred using two forks, season with salt and pepper, and return the chicken to the slow cooker.

5. Add the cream cheese, cover, and cook for 1 hour, stirring occasionally to make sure the cream cheese is melting and combined.

6. To serve, top with the avocado slices, sour cream, and shredded cheese (if using).

Make It Paleo: Check out my paleo-friendly Dairy-Free Cream Cheese (page 258) and Dairy-Free Sour Cream (page 259) recipes.

MACRONUTRIENTS	58% FAT	31% PROTEIN	11% CARBS

CALORIES: 325; TOTAL FAT: 21G; PROTEIN: 25G; TOTAL CARBS: 9G; FIBER: 2G; NET CARBS: 7G

BACON CHEESEBURGER SOUP

PREP TIME: 10 MINUTES **COOK TIME:** 40 MINUTES

In my last cookbook I gave you the Bacon Cheeseburger Casserole, and now here is a soup version! This soup is super filling, and anyone who loves cheeseburgers will love it—kids included! *Serves 4*

○ COMFORT FOOD
● NUT-FREE
● PALEO OR PALEO-FRIENDLY

3 bacon slices

6 ounces ground beef

Salt

Freshly ground black pepper

2 tablespoons butter or ghee

1 teaspoon chili powder

½ teaspoon garlic powder

½ teaspoon onion powder

2 cups beef broth or beef bone broth

1 teaspoon yellow mustard

½ cup shredded Cheddar cheese

2 pickle spears, diced

2 tablespoons tomato sauce or paste

2 ounces cream cheese or Dairy-Free Cream Cheese (page 258), cubed

¼ cup heavy whipping cream or full-fat unsweetened coconut milk

1. In a large skillet over medium-high heat, cook the bacon on both sides until crispy, about 8 minutes. Transfer the bacon to a paper towel–lined plate to drain and cool, then crumble it.

2. In the same skillet, add the ground beef to the bacon grease and season with salt and pepper. Stir occasionally, breaking the beef chunks apart. Cook for about 8 minutes, until browned.

3. Meanwhile, heat a pot or large saucepan over medium heat. Melt the butter and add the chili powder, garlic powder, and onion powder. Then add the beef broth, mustard, cheese, pickles, and tomato sauce. Cook for 5 to 10 minutes.

4. Adjust the heat to low and add the ground beef and cream cheese to the pot. Cover the pot and simmer on low for 20 minutes.

5. Turn off the heat and stir in the heavy cream.

6. Serve, topping each bowl with the crumbled bacon.

Make It Paleo: You can switch out the three dairy elements with dairy-free options to make this dish paleo-friendly. Use the Dairy-Free Cream Cheese recipe (page 258).

MACRONUTRIENTS	75% FAT	20% PROTEIN	5% CARBS

CALORIES: 410; TOTAL FAT: 34G; PROTEIN: 21G; TOTAL CARBS: 5G; FIBER: 1G; NET CARBS: 4G

CHICKEN COCONUT CURRY SOUP

PREP TIME: 10 MINUTES **COOK TIME:** 7 HOURS

I love a slow cooker soup. It makes you feel so accomplished when you come home to delicious smells and a simmering dish sitting there waiting for you! You can eat this as is or serve it over cauliflower rice—both ways are fantastic. (If you plan to serve it over cauliflower rice, you can leave the cauliflower florets out of the soup.) *Serves 4*

○ COMFORT FOOD

◐ DAIRY-FREE

● NUT-FREE

● PALEO OR PALEO-FRIENDLY

2 tablespoons butter or ghee

½ onion, diced

1 garlic clove, minced

1 teaspoon peeled, grated fresh ginger

1 teaspoon curry powder

1 teaspoon ground cumin

¼ teaspoon garam masala

Salt

Freshly ground black pepper

1 (13.5-ounce) can unsweetened full-fat coconut milk

1 cup vegetable broth, chicken broth, or chicken bone broth

½ cauliflower head, cut into florets

2 to 3 boneless chicken breasts

½ cup sliced mushrooms

2 tablespoons chopped cilantro

Lime wedges

1. In a skillet, melt the butter over medium heat. Add the onion and sauté, stirring occasionally, until softened.

2. Add the garlic, ginger, curry powder, cumin, and garam masala. Season with salt and pepper, and stir for about 30 seconds.

3. Remove the skillet from the heat and add the coconut milk and vegetable broth. Mix well.

4. In the slow cooker, arrange the cauliflower florets and chicken breasts. Pour the mixture from the skillet over the top of the chicken and cauliflower.

5. Cover and cook on low for 6½ hours.

6. Remove the chicken breasts, shred them with two forks, and season with salt and pepper before returning the shredded chicken back to the slow cooker. Add the sliced mushrooms.

7. Cover and cook for an additional 30 minutes and then serve.

8. Top the bowls with cilantro and serve with lime wedges.

Variation: You can easily switch out the chicken for shrimp. Just add the shrimp to the slow cooker for the last 15 minutes.

MACRONUTRIENTS	66% FAT	24% PROTEIN	10% CARBS

CALORIES: 410; TOTAL FAT: 30G; PROTEIN: 25G; TOTAL CARBS: 10G; FIBER: 2G; NET CARBS: 8G

CHICKEN TORTILLA SOUP

PREP TIME: 10 MINUTES **COOK TIME:** 8 HOURS

The only differences between my chicken tortilla soup and the regular, higher-carb, version is that I use low-carb tortillas, bake my own strips, and omit the corn. *Serves 4*

○ COMFORT FOOD
◐ DAIRY-FREE
● NUT-FREE
● PALEO OR PALEO-FRIENDLY

3 cups chicken broth or chicken bone broth

2 to 3 boneless chicken breasts

½ (15-ounce) can diced tomatoes with Italian seasoning

½ onion, diced

1 green bell pepper, diced

2 jalapeño peppers, seeded and minced

½ teaspoon chili powder

Salt

Freshly ground black pepper

1 low-carb tortilla, cut into ½-inch strips

1 tablespoon extra-virgin olive oil or avocado oil

1 teaspoon Tajín sauce

¼ cup shredded cheese (optional)

1 avocado, pitted, peeled, and cubed (optional)

2 tablespoons sour cream (optional)

1. In the slow cooker, combine the chicken broth, chicken breasts, tomatoes, onion, bell pepper, jalapeño peppers, and chili powder.

2. Cover and cook on low heat for 7 hours.

3. Remove the chicken breasts, shred with two forks, season with salt and pepper, and return the chicken to the slow cooker.

4. Cover and cook for 1 hour.

5. In the last 15 minutes, preheat the oven to 350°F.

6. On a baking sheet, arrange the tortilla strips in a single layer. Drizzle with the oil and season with salt and Tajín sauce. Bake for 8 to 10 minutes, until crisp.

7. Divide the soup into bowls and serve topped with the shredded cheese, avocado, and sour cream (if using).

Make Ahead: I usually make a double batch of this and eat it for days!

MACRONUTRIENTS	39% FAT	40% PROTEIN	21% CARBS

CALORIES: 251; TOTAL FAT: 11G; PROTEIN: 25G; TOTAL CARBS: 13G; FIBER: 3G; NET CARBS: 10G

MEDITERRANEAN WEDGE SALAD

PREP TIME: 10 MINUTES

A Mediterranean twist on a classic wedge salad came to me one day when I was out of romaine but had all of the ingredients to make a Greek salad. So I figured, why not wedge the iceberg? I'm so glad I did. *Serves 2*

- ● ALLERGEN-FREE
- ○ COMFORT FOOD
- ● DAIRY-FREE
- ● NUT-FREE
- ● PALEO OR PALEO-FRIENDLY
- ○ SUPER QUICK

½ cup grape tomatoes, halved

1 cucumber, diced

½ cup black olives, pitted and halved

1 teaspoon Italian Seasoning (page 246)

2 tablespoons extra-virgin olive oil, divided

Salt

Freshly ground black pepper

½ head iceberg lettuce, halved

1. In a medium bowl, combine the tomatoes, cucumber, olives, Italian seasoning, and 1 tablespoon of olive oil. Season with salt and pepper and toss.

2. Place a wedge of lettuce on each plate.

3. Top with the tomato, cucumber, and olive mixture. Drizzle the remaining 1 tablespoon of olive oil on top and add another pinch of salt.

Variation: Feta is a great addition; just sprinkle it on top. Also, if you like onions, you can add them to the tomato mixture.

MACRONUTRIENTS	75% FAT	3% PROTEIN	22% CARBS

CALORIES: 196; TOTAL FAT: 17G; PROTEIN: 2G; TOTAL CARBS: 12G; FIBER: 3G; NET CARBS: 9G

CREAMY CUCUMBER SALAD

PREP TIME: 5 MINUTES

I love cucumbers—they are so refreshing. This salad capitalizes on their flavor and texture, and could not be easier to make. It takes just 5 minutes and is amazing on a hot day. *Serves 2*

● NUT-FREE
○ SUPER QUICK

¼ cup sour cream

1 garlic clove, minced

1 lemon wedge, juiced

2 cucumbers, diced

4 radishes, sliced thin

Salt

Freshly ground black pepper

2 tablespoons chopped fresh dill

1. In a small bowl, mix the sour cream, garlic, and lemon juice.

2. In a large bowl, toss the cucumbers and radishes, and season with salt and pepper. Pour the sour cream dressing over the vegetables and toss.

3. Top with the dill and serve.

Variation: I am not a huge fan of onions, but if you are, you can add ½ red onion, thinly sliced.

MACRONUTRIENTS	46% FAT	10% PROTEIN	44% CARBS

CALORIES: 118; TOTAL FAT: 6G; PROTEIN: 3G; TOTAL CARBS: 13G; FIBER: 2G; NET CARBS: 11G

AVOCADO COTIJA SALAD

PREP TIME: 5 MINUTES

This is one of my favorite salads to make when I have people coming over. It is super simple and everyone (keto or not) loves it! If you have never tried cotija cheese, you must! It is crumbly, salty, and delicious. *Serves 2*

● NUT-FREE
○ SUPER QUICK

2 tablespoons extra-virgin olive oil

1 tablespoon freshly squeezed lime juice

2 cucumbers, diced

2 avocados, pitted, peeled, and diced

½ cup grape tomatoes, halved

¼ cup crumbled cotija cheese or feta cheese

¼ cup chopped fresh mint

1. In a small bowl, whisk together the olive oil and lime juice.

2. In a large bowl, toss the cucumbers, avocados, and tomatoes, and season with salt and pepper. Pour the dressing over the cucumber mixture and toss to combine.

3. Add the cotija cheese and fresh mint, and toss again.

Variation: To add a little spice, add 1 diced jalapeño pepper with the ribs and seeds removed.

MACRONUTRIENTS	74% FAT	6% PROTEIN	20% CARBS

CALORIES: 454; TOTAL FAT: 39G; PROTEIN: 8G; TOTAL CARBS: 27G; FIBER: 12G; NET CARBS: 15G

THAI SHRIMP AND ZOODLE SALAD

PREP TIME: 15 MINUTES **COOK TIME:** 10 MINUTES

Switch out your traditional greens with zoodles (zucchini noodles) in this salad for a fresh, crunchy twist! Grab your spiralizer or, if you're like me, buy prespiralized zoodles at your grocery store. *Serves 2*

○ COMFORT FOOD
◐ DAIRY-FREE
● NUT-FREE
● PALEO OR PALEO-FRIENDLY
○ SUPER QUICK

2 zucchini, spiralized (zoodles)

Salt

8 ounces peeled shrimp

¼ teaspoon paprika

2 tablespoons extra-virgin olive oil or ghee, divided

2 garlic cloves, minced

½ (15-ounce) can diced tomatoes with Italian seasoning

¼ teaspoon red pepper flakes

½ cup black olives, sliced

Freshly ground black pepper

¼ cup chopped fresh basil

1. Place the zoodles on a paper towel–lined plate and season with salt.

2. In a small bowl, season the shrimp with salt and the paprika.

3. In a skillet, heat 1 tablespoon of olive oil over medium-high heat. Add the shrimp and cook for about 2 minutes on each side. Set aside on a plate.

4. Reduce the heat to medium and add the remaining 1 tablespoon of olive oil. Cook the garlic until softened.

5. Add the tomatoes, red pepper flakes, and olives. Season with salt and pepper and heat until the mixture simmers.

6. Add the zoodles to the sauce and simmer for 2 minutes.

7. Add the shrimp and toss everything well.

8. Divide between two bowls and top with the basil.

Variation: If you eat dairy, you can add ½ cup of Alfredo sauce to the diced tomato mixture for a take on a rosa Alfredo sauce and for some added fat.

MACRONUTRIENTS	51% FAT	33% PROTEIN	16% CARBS

CALORIES: 335; TOTAL FAT: 19G; PROTEIN: 28G; TOTAL CARBS: 13G; FIBER: 4G; NET CARBS: 9G

ANTIPASTO SALAD

PREP TIME: 10 MINUTES

Every time I go to an Italian restaurant, I end up ordering the antipasto salad. I like to make my own version at home, as well. It's full of flavor, and you can get creative with your ingredients. This is also a simple salad to throw together for a large group, or to break up for multiple lunches if you like to do meal prep. *Serves 2*

○ COMFORT FOOD
◐ DAIRY-FREE
● NUT-FREE
● PALEO OR PALEO-FRIENDLY
○ SUPER QUICK

1 head romaine lettuce, finely chopped

6 pepperoncini peppers, sliced

¼ cup uncured pepperoni, cut into strips

¼ cup uncured salami, cut into strips

½ cup artichoke hearts, drained and halved

¼ cup black olives, sliced

¼ cup green olives, sliced

2 tablespoons grated Parmesan cheese (optional)

1 tablespoon paleo-friendly vinaigrette or Italian dressing

In a large bowl, combine the romaine, pepperoncini peppers, pepperoni, salami, artichoke hearts, black olives, green olives, Parmesan (if using), and vinaigrette. Combine all the ingredients and toss.

Variation: Toasted pine nuts make a great addition. Heat a dry skillet over medium-low heat and add the pine nuts. You need to stir the pine nuts frequently to brown them evenly; be careful not to burn them. It should take 2½ to 3 minutes.

MACRONUTRIENTS	67% FAT	14% PROTEIN	19% CARBS

CALORIES: 240; TOTAL FAT: 18G; PROTEIN: 9G; TOTAL CARBS: 14G; FIBER: 8G; NET CARBS: 6G

CHOPPED BUFFALO CHICKEN SALAD

PREP TIME: 10 MINUTES

This recipe brings all the flavors of buffalo wings into a salad! It's easy to pull together, and I love making this meal when I have leftover chicken breasts. *Serves 2*

● NUT-FREE
○ SUPER QUICK

1 cooked chicken breast, cubed

2 tablespoons hot sauce, divided

1 head romaine lettuce, finely chopped

1 cucumber, chopped

1 avocado, pitted, peeled, and diced

½ cup chopped celery

¼ cup blue cheese crumbles (optional)

2 tablespoons paleo-friendly ranch dressing

1. In a small bowl, toss the chicken with 1 tablespoon of hot sauce.

2. In a large bowl, combine the romaine, cucumber, avocado, and celery, and toss.

3. Add the chicken and blue cheese crumbles (if using) to the vegetables and toss again.

4. In a small bowl, mix the ranch dressing with the remaining 1 tablespoon of hot sauce and drizzle over the salad.

Make It Paleo: Leave off the blue cheese crumbles. The ranch I use is made with avocado oil and is paleo-compliant.

MACRONUTRIENTS	46% FAT	32% PROTEIN	22% CARBS

CALORIES: 336; TOTAL FAT: 18G; PROTEIN: 27G; TOTAL CARBS: 21G; FIBER: 11G; NET CARBS: 10G

CRUNCHY THAI CHICKEN SALAD

PREP TIME: 20 MINUTES

This combination of crunchy cabbage and peanuts with creamy peanut butter sauce is divine. Most restaurant versions of this salad are loaded with sugar, but not this one. Use a peanut butter or nut butter without added sugar. (Personally I love peanut butter, so I eat it in small amounts, but some people on keto don't eat peanuts at all since they are a legume.) *Serves 2*

○ DAIRY-FREE
○ SUPER QUICK

FOR THE PEANUT SAUCE DRESSING

2 tablespoons peanut butter or nut butter

1 tablespoon coconut aminos or soy sauce

1 teaspoon sesame oil

¼ teaspoon Sriracha

FOR THE SALAD

1 cooked chicken breast, shredded

2 tablespoons peanuts, chopped

1 cup shredded mixed-colors cabbage

¼ cup chopped broccoli

2 tablespoons sliced scallions, green parts only

2 tablespoons chopped cilantro

1 cucumber, diced

1 tablespoon freshly squeezed lime juice

TO MAKE THE PEANUT SAUCE DRESSING

In a blender or food processor, combine the peanut butter, coconut aminos, sesame oil, and Sriracha, and process until smooth.

TO MAKE THE SALAD

In a large bowl, toss the chicken, peanuts, cabbage, broccoli, scallions, cilantro, and cucumber. Serve topped with the peanut sauce dressing and lime juice.

Make Ahead: This salad works great for meal prep. Just wait to toss with the dressing until right before eating.

MACRONUTRIENTS	47% FAT	38% PROTEIN	15% CARBS

CALORIES: 354; TOTAL FAT: 18G; PROTEIN: 38G; TOTAL CARBS: 12G; FIBER: 4G; NET CARBS: 8G

BACON-STRAWBERRY SPINACH SALAD

PREP TIME: 5 MINUTES **COOK TIME:** 8 MINUTES

Berries are a keto-approved fruit, so I love to incorporate them into my diet a couple of times a week. It doesn't take a lot to add a refreshing sweetness, and just two strawberries really complement the fat in the bacon and avocado. *Serves 2*

● ALLERGEN-FREE
○ COMFORT FOOD
◐ DAIRY-FREE
● NUT-FREE
● PALEO OR PALEO-FRIENDLY
○ SUPER QUICK

6 bacon slices

2 tablespoons extra-virgin olive oil

1 tablespoon freshly squeezed lemon juice

4 cups spinach

2 strawberries, sliced

1 avocado, pitted, peeled, and diced

Salt

Freshly ground black pepper

1. In a large skillet over medium-high heat, cook the bacon on both sides until crispy, about 8 minutes. Transfer to a paper towel–lined plate to drain and cool, then crumble it.

2. In a small bowl, whisk together the olive oil and lemon juice.

3. In a large bowl, toss the spinach, bacon, strawberries, and avocado. Season with salt and pepper.

4. Drizzle the dressing on top and stir to combine. Serve.

MACRONUTRIENTS	79% FAT	12% PROTEIN	9% CARBS

CALORIES: 380; TOTAL FAT: 34G; PROTEIN: 12G; TOTAL CARBS: 10G; FIBER: 6G; NET CARBS: 4G

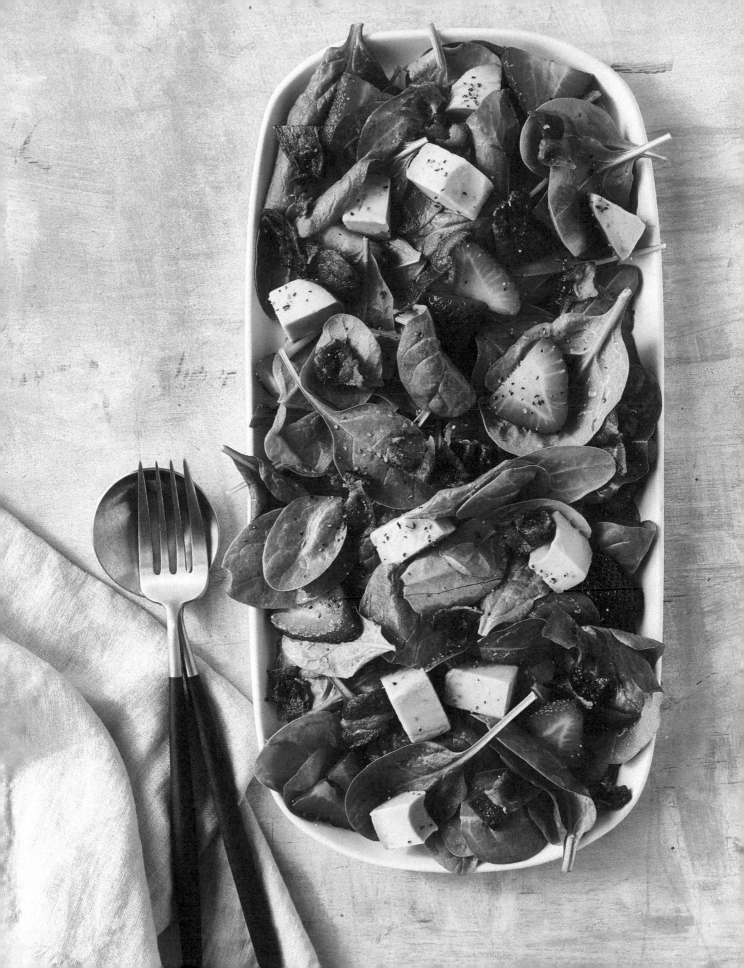

BAE (BACON, AVOCADO, EGG) BUTTER LETTUCE SALAD

PREP TIME: 15 MINUTES **COOK TIME:** 20 MINUTES

A restaurant near my office makes this eggs and bacon butter lettuce salad, which I love. One weekend I was home and started craving it, so I whipped up my own. *Serves 2*

○ COMFORT FOOD

◐ DAIRY-FREE

● NUT-FREE

● PALEO OR PALEO-FRIENDLY

2 large eggs

4 bacon slices

1 small head butter lettuce

½ tablespoon extra-virgin olive oil

Salt

Freshly ground black pepper

1 avocado, pitted, peeled, and diced

½ teaspoon freshly squeezed lemon or lime juice

1. In a small saucepan, cover the eggs with water and cook over high heat. Once the water is boiling, turn off the heat, cover, and leave on the burner for 10 to 12 minutes.

2. While the eggs are cooking, heat a large skillet over medium-high heat. Cook the bacon on both sides until crispy, about 8 minutes. Transfer the bacon to a paper towel–lined plate to drain and cool, then crumble it.

3. Separate the butter lettuce leaves, wash, and pat dry. Divide the leaves between two plates and drizzle the olive oil over them. Season with a pinch of salt and pepper.

4. Peel and chop the hard-boiled eggs and put them in a bowl. Add the avocado and, using a fork, mash the egg and avocado together. Season with salt and pepper, add the lemon juice, and stir to combine.

5. Place an even scoop of the egg-avocado mixture in the middle of each salad. Sprinkle the bacon on top.

Allergen Tip: You can leave out the egg in this salad and instead use ¼ cup of diced tofu to mix in with the avocado.

MACRONUTRIENTS	72% FAT	18% PROTEIN	10% CARBS

CALORIES: 313; TOTAL FAT: 26G; PROTEIN: 15G; TOTAL CARBS: 9G; FIBER: 6G; NET CARBS: 3G

CHILI-LIME SHRIMP COBB SALAD

PREP TIME: 10 MINUTES **COOK TIME:** 20 MINUTES

You can't really have a keto cookbook and not have a Cobb salad recipe; it's basically the perfect keto food! But for some reason, I just do not get excited about Cobb salads with turkey—it's just so blah. In my last book, I had a Cobb salad with skirt steak and one with salmon. Now I'm offering this shrimp version. The shrimp in this recipe is seasoned with yummy Chili-Lime Seasoning (page 244) for a kick. Enjoy! *Serves 2*

○ COMFORT FOOD
○ SUPER QUICK

½ pound shrimp, peeled and deveined

2 tablespoons extra-virgin olive oil, divided

1 tablespoon Chili-Lime Seasoning (page 244)

Salt

Freshly ground black pepper

2 large eggs

4 bacon slices

3 cups chopped romaine lettuce

1 teaspoon freshly squeezed lemon juice

1 avocado, pitted, peeled, and diced

¼ cup pecans, roughly chopped

¼ cup crumbled goat cheese (optional)

1. Preheat the oven to 400°F. Line a baking sheet with parchment paper or a silicone baking mat.

2. In a medium bowl, toss the shrimp with 1 tablespoon of olive oil and the chili-lime seasoning. Season with salt and pepper. Transfer the shrimp to a baking sheet in a single layer and cook for 5 minutes.

3. In a small saucepan, cover the eggs with water and cook over high heat. Once the water is boiling, turn off the heat, cover, and leave on the burner for 10 to 12 minutes.

4. While the eggs are cooking, heat a large skillet over medium-high heat, and cook the bacon on both sides until crispy, about 8 minutes. Transfer the bacon to a paper towel–lined plate to drain and cool, then crumble it.

5. Divide the romaine between two bowls, drizzle with the remaining 1 tablespoon of olive oil and the lemon juice, and season with salt and pepper.

6. Peel and chop the hard-boiled eggs.

7. Assemble the salads by arranging the toppings of shrimp, eggs, avocado, pecans, bacon, and goat cheese (if using), each in its own section. You can do thick stripes of the ingredients, or divide them like a pie.

Make It Paleo: Just leave off the goat cheese to make this paleo-friendly.

MACRONUTRIENTS	67% FAT	26% PROTEIN	7% CARBS

CALORIES: 741; TOTAL FAT: 53G; PROTEIN: 52G; TOTAL CARBS: 14G; FIBER: 8G; NET CARBS: 6G

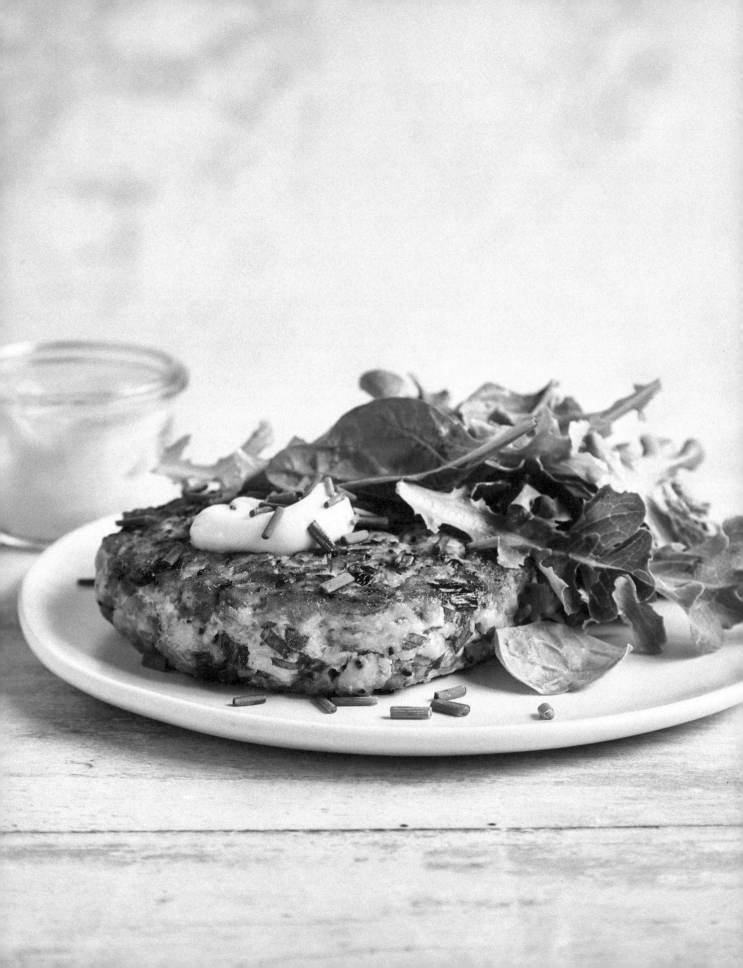

FISH

CHAPTER EIGHT

Opposite: Salmon Burgers with Chive Aioli and Greens

SALMON BURGERS
WITH CHIVE AIOLI AND GREENS

PREP TIME: 10 MINUTES **COOK TIME:** 10 MINUTES

Salmon is one of my favorite foods, raw or cooked. Salmon burgers in particular are a fun way to mix it up since they take on flavors really well. The creamy aioli sauce adds deliciousness. *Serves 2*

○ COMFORT FOOD
◐ DAIRY-FREE
● NUT-FREE
○ SUPER QUICK

¼ cup pork rinds

12 ounces ground salmon*

1 bunch scallions, sliced, green parts only

1 tablespoon capers

1 tablespoon prepared horseradish

1 tablespoon Dijon mustard

Salt

Freshly ground black pepper

1 tablespoon cooking oil or ghee

6 ounces mixed greens

1 tablespoon MCT oil or Brain Octane Oil, divided

2 tablespoons avocado oil mayonnaise

Chopped fresh chives, for garnish

1. In a food processor, pulse the pork rinds until they are a bread crumb consistency.

2. In a large mixing bowl, combine the salmon, scallions, capers, horseradish, Dijon, and pork rinds. Season with salt and pepper. Mix with your hands and create two 1-inch-thick burgers. Transfer the burgers to a plate and refrigerate for 10 minutes.

3. Heat a skillet or grill pan on medium heat. Add the cooking oil, and once it is simmering, add the burgers.

4. Cook on each side for 4 to 5 minutes, flipping once.

5. Divide the greens between two plates and toss with the MCT oil. Season with salt and pepper.

6. Place the cooked burgers on top of the greens and top them with the mayonnaise and a sprinkle of chives.

Note: I prefer to use chunks of raw salmon, which can usually be found in the seafood section of specialty markets, but it is fine to use 2 cans of cooked, canned salmon (found near the canned tuna) instead.

MACRONUTRIENTS	59% FAT	32% PROTEIN	9% CARBS

CALORIES: 471; TOTAL FAT: 31G; PROTEIN: 38G; TOTAL CARBS: 10G; FIBER: 2G; NET CARBS: 8G

POACHED SALMON
WITH CREAMY CUCUMBER SAUCE

PREP TIME: 10 MINUTES **COOK TIME:** 7 MINUTES

I could probably eat salmon every single day. This version is poached, and I love the fresh, creamy cucumber sauce because it adds fat and flavor. There's nothing quite like the tang of sour cream with a lovely pop of dill. *Serves 2*

● NUT-FREE
○ SUPER QUICK

1 small cucumber, diced

½ cup sour cream

¼ teaspoon white wine vinegar, plus 3 tablespoons

1 teaspoon salt, plus more for seasoning

2 (4-ounce) salmon fillets, skin on

2 tablespoons fresh dill

1. In a small bowl, toss the cucumber, sour cream, and ¼ teaspoon vinegar. Season with salt and mix thoroughly. Place in the refrigerator to chill while the salmon cooks.

2. Fill a wide saucepan with 3 inches of water, the remaining 3 tablespoons of vinegar, and 1 teaspoon of salt. Bring to a boil.

3. Add the salmon to the pan, skin-side down. Cook for 5 to 7 minutes. (I like my salmon on the medium-rare side, so 5 minutes works for me.) You want the outer skin to be opaque.

4. Using a slotted spoon, remove the salmon and place it on a paper towel–lined plate to absorb any excess water.

5. Remove the cucumber sauce from the refrigerator and gently stir in the dill.

6. Plate the salmon and add the cucumber sauce on top of each fillet.

Make It Paleo: You can use the Dairy-Free Sour Cream (page 259).

MACRONUTRIENTS	57% FAT	35% PROTEIN	8% CARBS

CALORIES: 291; TOTAL FAT: 19G; PROTEIN: 24G; TOTAL CARBS: 6G; FIBER: 1G; NET CARBS: 5G

SPICY SHRIMP WITH SHIRATAKI NOODLES

PREP TIME: 10 MINUTES **COOK TIME:** 10 MINUTES

Shirataki noodles are so easy to make and allow you turn your previously carb-filled pasta recipes into keto-friendly meals. The spicy marinara-style sauce in this recipe coats the noodles and is so good that I could eat it straight with a spoon. *Serves 2*

○ COMFORT FOOD
◐ DAIRY-FREE
● NUT-FREE
● PALEO OR PALEO-FRIENDLY
○ SUPER QUICK

6 ounces shrimp, peeled

Salt

¼ teaspoon paprika

2 tablespoons extra-virgin olive oil, avocado oil, or ghee, divided

2 garlic cloves, minced

6 ounces crushed tomatoes

¼ teaspoon red pepper flakes

Freshly ground black pepper

¼ cup chopped fresh basil

1 batch Shirataki Noodles (page 40)

1. In a small bowl, season the shrimp with salt and the paprika.

2. In a skillet over medium heat, add 1 tablespoon of oil and when it is hot, add the shrimp. Cook for 2 minutes per side. Remove the shrimp from the skillet and set aside on a plate.

3. Add the remaining 1 tablespoon of oil and cook the garlic for about 1 minute, until soft.

4. Add the tomatoes and red pepper flakes, season with salt and pepper, and stir. Heat until the tomatoes begin to lightly boil.

5. Reduce the heat to low and add the basil and shrimp. Simmer on low for 2 minutes.

6. Serve the shrimp on top of the shirataki noodles.

Variation: You can also use zoodles (zucchini noodles) in this dish if you prefer. If you're using zoodles, cook them per the directions on page 37. You can buy them prespiralized at many grocery stores or you can spiralize two zucchini yourself.

MACRONUTRIENTS	56% FAT	32% PROTEIN	12% CARBS

CALORIES: 240; TOTAL FAT: 15G; PROTEIN: 19G; TOTAL CARBS: 8G; FIBER: 2G; NET CARBS: 6G

SPICY TUNA POKE BOWL

PREP TIME: 5 MINUTES, PLUS 20 MINUTES TO MARINATE

I love this easy spin on poke and its great use of avocado. (Finding new ways to use avocado as a vessel for yummy flavors is always fun.) The other great thing about this recipe is that raw fish means no cooking, so you can have this delicious meal ready in minutes! *Serves 2*

○ COMFORT FOOD
◐ DAIRY-FREE
● NUT-FREE
● PALEO OR PALEO-FRIENDLY
○ SUPER QUICK

10 ounces sushi-grade ahi tuna, cubed

1 tablespoon sesame oil

1 tablespoon coconut aminos or soy sauce

1 tablespoon freshly squeezed lime juice

½ tablespoon lime zest

1 teaspoon peeled, grated fresh ginger

Freshly ground black pepper

1 tablespoon avocado mayonnaise

1 tablespoon Sriracha

2 avocados, halved and pitted

1 tablespoon sesame seeds or furikake

1 tablespoon chopped fresh chives

1. Rinse the tuna in cold water and pat dry. Cut into cubes and place in a medium mixing bowl.

2. In the same bowl, add the sesame oil, coconut aminos, lime juice, lime zest, and ginger. Season with pepper. Mix to coat and then place in the refrigerator for 10 to 20 minutes to marinate.

3. In a small bowl, mix the mayonnaise and Sriracha. If you like spice, you can add more Sriracha.

4. Remove the tuna from the refrigerator and spoon the mixture into the avocado halves.

5. Drizzle the Sriracha mayonnaise on top, and garnish with the sesame seeds and chives.

Variation: Traditionally, poke is served in a bowl with rice. If you prefer, you can cube the avocado and place all of the ingredients on top of a keto-friendly base, like fresh mixed greens, shirataki rice, or cauliflower rice.

MACRONUTRIENTS	59% FAT	28% PROTEIN	13% CARBS

CALORIES: 518; TOTAL FAT: 34G; PROTEIN: 37G; TOTAL CARBS: 16G; FIBER: 10G; NET CARBS: 6G

SHRIMP SCAMPI WITH ZOODLES

PREP TIME: 10 MINUTES **COOK TIME:** 15 MINUTES

The smell of butter and garlic is one of my favorites. I love the way it fills the house. I consider shrimp scampi a comfort food, and it's also very easy to make but always looks really impressive. This version uses zoodles (zucchini noodles) to keep it keto-friendly. *Serves 2*

○ COMFORT FOOD
● NUT-FREE
○ SUPER QUICK

3 tablespoons butter or ghee

2 garlic cloves, minced

1 shallot, thinly sliced

12 ounces shrimp, peeled and deveined

¼ teaspoon red pepper flakes

½ lemon, juiced

1 tablespoon minced fresh parsley

2 zucchini, spiralized (zoodles)

Salt

Freshly ground black pepper

¼ cup grated Parmesan cheese

1. In a large skillet, melt the butter over medium heat. Add the garlic and shallot and sauté until softened.

2. In a small bowl, season the shrimp with the red pepper flakes and add to the skillet. Cook for about 1 minute and flip.

3. Once the second side is almost done, about 1 minute more, add the lemon juice. Reduce the heat slightly, then turn it off. Add the parsley and zoodles, and toss.

4. Season the scampi with salt and pepper. Divide between two plates and top with the Parmesan cheese.

Variation: Try adding veggies like cherry tomatoes, asparagus, or fresh spinach to your scampi. You can also add white wine at the same time as the lemon juice.

MACRONUTRIENTS	52% FAT	43% PROTEIN	5% CARBS

CALORIES: 397; TOTAL FAT: 24G; PROTEIN: 40G; TOTAL CARBS: 5G; FIBER: 0G; NET CARBS: 5G

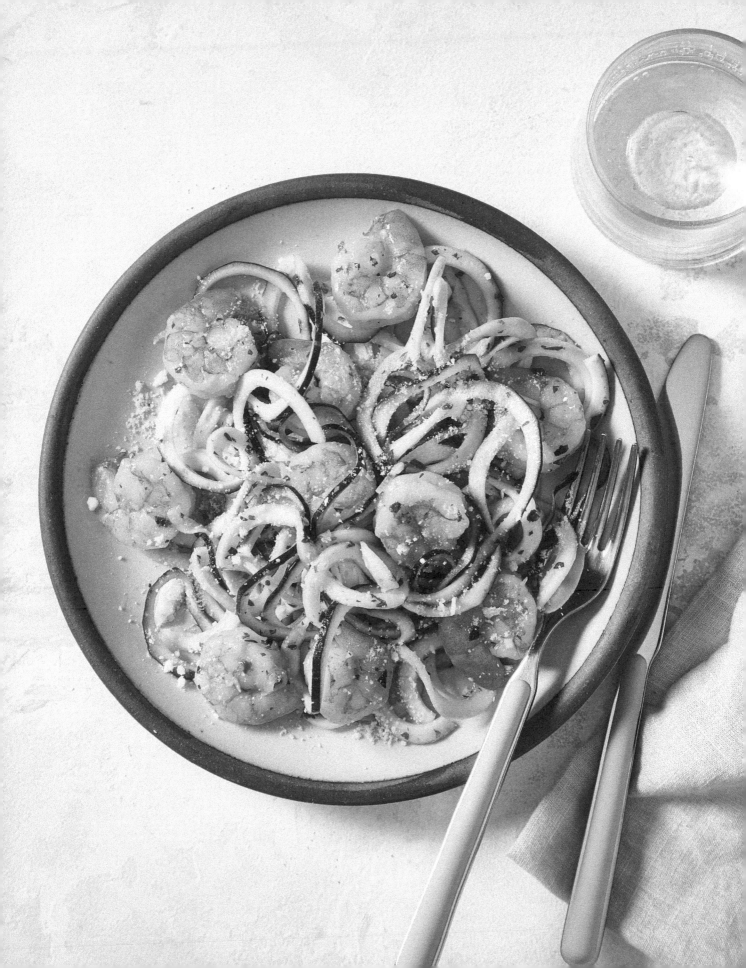

BACON AND JALAPEÑO WRAPPED SHRIMP

PREP TIME: 10 MINUTES **COOK TIME:** 20 MINUTES

You might think cheese and shrimp is a strange combo, but I promise you will love it. Here the combo is paired with bacon and jalapeño peppers for a dish that is packed with flavor and makes a great party appetizer or dinner. *Serves 2*

● NUT-FREE
○ SUPER QUICK

4 jalapeño peppers, seeded and cut into 3 to 4 long strips each

12 large shrimp, deveined, butterflied, tail-on

Salt

Freshly ground black pepper

6 thin bacon slices

¼ cup shredded pepper jack cheese

1. Preheat the oven to 350°F.

2. On a baking sheet, arrange the jalapeño strips in a single layer and roast for 10 minutes.

3. In a small bowl, season the shrimp with salt and pepper.

4. Remove the jalapeño strips from the oven. Place a strip inside each open butterflied shrimp. Wrap each shrimp with bacon and secure with a toothpick. Arrange in a single layer on a baking sheet.

5. Cook for 8 minutes, until the bacon is crispy.

6. Adjust the oven to broil.

7. Sprinkle the cheese on top of the shrimp and broil for about 1 minute, until the cheese is bubbling.

Make It Paleo: Skip the cheese and dip these in Sriracha mayonnaise for an added creamy element.

MACRONUTRIENTS	58% FAT	38% PROTEIN	4% CARBS

CALORIES: 240; TOTAL FAT: 16G; PROTEIN: 21G; TOTAL CARBS: 3G; FIBER: 1G; NET CARBS: 2G

CRISPY FISH STICKS

PREP TIME: 10 MINUTES **COOK TIME:** 10 MINUTES

I wanted to find a way to make a keto-friendly version of fish sticks that both kids and adults would love. Fish sticks always remind me of my childhood. I think it was probably the only seafood my mom cooked when I was growing up! Now I eat seafood at least four days a week, but I still can't get enough of these things. *Serves 4*

○ COMFORT FOOD
○ SUPER QUICK

1 cup avocado oil or other cooking oil, plus more as needed

1 pound frozen cod, thawed

2 large eggs

2 tablespoons avocado oil mayonnaise

1 cup almond flour

½ cup grated Parmesan cheese

½ cup ground pork rinds

½ teaspoon chili powder

½ teaspoon chopped fresh parsley

Salt

Freshly ground black pepper

¼ cup Dairy-Free Tartar Sauce (page 253)

1. In a skillet, heat the avocado oil over high heat. You want the oil to be about ½ inch deep, so adjust the amount of oil based on the size of your pan.

2. Pat the fish dry with paper towels to remove any excess water.

3. In a small bowl, whisk the eggs and mayonnaise together.

4. In another bowl, combine the almond flour, Parmesan, pork rinds, chili powder, and parsley. Season with salt and pepper.

5. Cut the cod into strips.

6. Dip the fish into the egg mixture and then dredge in the dry mixture. Press the strips into the dry mixture so that the "breading" sticks well on all sides.

7. Add 3 to 4 fish sticks at a time to the hot oil. The oil should sizzle when you add the fish sticks. Cook for 2 minutes per side, or until golden and crispy.

8. Place the cooked fish sticks on a paper towel–lined plate while you continue to fry the rest of the fish sticks.

9. Serve with the tartar sauce on the side.

Variation: If you don't have pork rinds on hand, you can skip them and double up on the Parmesan cheese.

MACRONUTRIENTS	67% FAT	30% PROTEIN	3% CARBS (NOT INCLUDING COOKING OIL)

CALORIES: 402; TOTAL FAT: 30G; PROTEIN: 30G; TOTAL CARBS: 3G; FIBER: 1G; NET CARBS: 2G

PROSCIUTTO-WRAPPED COD

PREP TIME: 5 MINUTES **COOK TIME:** 10 MINUTES

In my opinion, prosciutto is good wrapped around just about anything, but I especially love this dish because the prosciutto gets crispy and becomes a great contrast to the soft, flaky fish. Note that I do not season the fish with salt in this recipe because prosciutto is very salty on its own. *Serves 2*

○ COMFORT FOOD
◐ DAIRY-FREE
● NUT-FREE
● PALEO OR PALEO-FRIENDLY
○ SUPER QUICK

2 (6-ounce) cod fillets

Freshly ground black pepper

4 prosciutto slices

2 tablespoons butter or ghee

1. Pat the fish dry with paper towels to remove any excess water.

2. Season the fillets with pepper and wrap the prosciutto around the fillets.

3. Heat a skillet over medium heat and add the butter.

4. Once the pan is hot, add the fillets and cook on each side for 5 minutes, or until the outside is crispy and the inside is flaky.

5. Place the cooked fish onto a paper towel–lined plate to absorb any excess oil.

Variation: You can replace the cod with another white fish if you'd prefer. (Wild-caught fish is always best if you can get it.) This dish also pairs wonderfully with the Lemony Spinach (page 210).

MACRONUTRIENTS	50% FAT	48% PROTEIN	2% CARBS

CALORIES: 317; TOTAL FAT: 18G; PROTEIN: 38G; TOTAL CARBS: 0G; FIBER: 0G; NET CARBS: 0G

COCONUT MAHI-MAHI NUGGETS

PREP TIME: 10 MINUTES **COOK TIME:** 10 MINUTES

Fish with a tropical twist! The combination of mahi-mahi, coconut, macadamia nuts, and lime is just stunning! I love macadamia nuts, so anything crusted with them is a winner in my book. *Serves 2*

○ COMFORT FOOD
◐ DAIRY-FREE
● PALEO OR PALEO-FRIENDLY
○ SUPER QUICK

1 cup avocado oil or coconut oil, plus more as needed

1 pound frozen mahi-mahi, thawed

2 large eggs

2 tablespoons avocado oil mayonnaise

1 cup almond flour

½ cup shredded coconut

¼ cup crushed macadamia nuts

Salt

Freshly ground black pepper

½ lime, cut into wedges

¼ cup Dairy-Free Tartar Sauce (page 253)

1. In a skillet, heat the avocado oil over high heat. You want the oil to be about ½ inch deep, so adjust the amount of oil based on the size of your pan.

2. Pat the fish dry with paper towels to remove any excess water.

3. In a small bowl, whisk the eggs and mayonnaise together.

4. In a medium mixing bowl, combine the almond flour, coconut, and macadamia nuts. Season with salt and pepper. Cut the mahi-mahi into nuggets.

5. Dip the fish into the egg mixture and then dredge in the dry mixture. Press into the dry mixture so that "breading" sticks well on all sides.

6. Add the fish into the hot oil. It should sizzle when you add the nuggets. Cook for 2 minutes per side, until golden and crispy. Depending on the size of your skillet, you can do all the nuggets at once or in two groups.

7. Place the cooked nuggets on a paper towel–lined plate and squirt the lime wedges over them.

Allergen Tip: If you are allergic to eggs, you can use a liquid egg replacement. The mayonnaise I use is also egg free and made with avocado oil.

MACRONUTRIENTS	65% FAT	29% PROTEIN	6% CARBS (NOT INCLUDING COOKING OIL)

CALORIES: 733; TOTAL FAT: 53G; PROTEIN: 54G; TOTAL CARBS: 10G; FIBER: 6G; NET CARBS: 4G

CREAMY GARLIC BUTTER SALMON

PREP TIME: 5 MINUTES **COOK TIME:** 20 MINUTES

This recipe is a winner because of the creamy, flavorful sauce prepared with my favorite fish, salmon. I love eating this dish with shirataki noodles, shirataki rice, or cauliflower rice. *Serves 2*

○ COMFORT FOOD
● NUT-FREE
○ SUPER QUICK

2 tablespoons extra-virgin olive oil, avocado oil, or ghee

2 salmon fillets

Salt

Freshly ground black pepper

2 tablespoons butter or ghee

3 garlic cloves, minced

½ small onion, diced

½ cup heavy whipping cream

3 cups fresh spinach

¼ cup grated Parmesan cheese

1 tablespoon chopped fresh parsley

1. In a skillet, heat the olive oil over medium-high heat.

2. Pat the salmon dry to remove any excess water and season with salt and pepper on both sides.

3. Sear the salmon on both sides, about 4 minutes per side. Transfer the salmon to a plate.

4. In the same skillet, melt the butter over medium heat. Add the garlic and onion and sauté until softened.

5. Reduce the heat to low and add the heavy cream. Bring to a simmer, whisking or stirring occasionally.

6. Add the whole leaves of spinach to the cream sauce and season with salt and pepper. Add the Parmesan cheese and simmer until the spinach wilts and the cheese melts.

7. Add the salmon back to pan, and spoon the sauce on top. Serve garnished with the parsley.

Variation: Whether you cook the salmon with the skin on or not is a personal preference, but salmon skin, especially from wild-caught Pacific salmon, has the highest concentration of omega-3 fatty acids.

MACRONUTRIENTS	77% FAT	19% PROTEIN	4% CARBS

CALORIES: 652; TOTAL FAT: 57G; PROTEIN: 29G; TOTAL CARBS: 7G; FIBER: 1G; NET CARBS: 6G

BROILED LOBSTER TAILS

PREP TIME: 10 MINUTES **COOK TIME:** 10 MINUTES

Lobster is such a luxury—it's so rich. It's also perfect for keto when you dip it in butter! I had never even attempted to cook lobster at home until a couple of years ago when I discovered how easy it is to broil lobster tails. Now this is something I love to cook. *Serves 2*

○ COMFORT FOOD

◐ DAIRY-FREE

● NUT-FREE

● PALEO OR PALEO-FRIENDLY

○ SUPER QUICK

2 lobster tails

½ lemon, cut into wedges

Salt

1 teaspoon paprika

1 teaspoon garlic powder

4 tablespoons butter or ghee, divided

1 teaspoon chopped fresh parsley

1. Preheat the broiler.

2. Using kitchen scissors, carefully cut the top of the lobster shell down the middle from the tip to the tail. Be sure not to cut the meat. If there's any grit, remove it now.

3. Open the shell. Squirt the lobster flesh with the juice from 1 lemon wedge and then place additional lemon wedges under the meat.

4. Season with salt and sprinkle the paprika and garlic powder on top of the lobster meat. Place 1 tablespoon of butter on top of each.

5. Place the lobster tails in a small casserole or on a baking sheet and broil for 10 minutes.

6. While the lobster is broiling, melt the remaining 2 tablespoons of butter in the microwave or on the stove top.

7. Remove the lobster from the broiler, add the parsley, and serve with the melted butter for dipping.

Variation: You can use frozen lobster tails, but be sure to place them in the refrigerator the day before cooking to thaw them.

MACRONUTRIENTS	73% FAT	25% PROTEIN	2% CARBS

CALORIES: 285; TOTAL FAT: 24G; PROTEIN: 17G; TOTAL CARBS: 2G; FIBER: 1G; NET CARBS: 1G

GARLIC CRAB LEGS

PREP TIME: 10 MINUTES **COOK TIME:** 20 MINUTES

I've learned that the way to my daughter's heart is through crab legs. She loves these in particular because they are garlicky and full of flavor. I love them because they could not be easier to make! I'm a big fan of king crab legs myself, but the problem is that I could eat crab forever without getting full, and that can get expensive! *Serves 2*

○ COMFORT FOOD
● NUT-FREE
● PALEO OR PALEO-FRIENDLY
○ SUPER QUICK

4 tablespoons butter or ghee

2 tablespoons extra-virgin olive oil

½ lemon, juiced and zested

4 garlic cloves, crushed and minced

2 teaspoons Old Bay Seasoning

1 tablespoon red pepper flakes

2 pounds crab legs

2 tablespoons chopped
fresh parsley

1. Preheat the oven to 375°F.

2. Heat a large oven-safe skillet over medium-low heat. Add the butter, olive oil, lemon juice, lemon zest, garlic, Old Bay, and red pepper flakes. Sauté for 2 minutes.

3. Add the crab legs and parsley to the skillet. Spoon the butter mixture over the crab and baste for 3 minutes.

4. Place the skillet in the oven and bake for 15 minutes, basting every 5 minutes.

5. Place the crab legs on a platter and pour the butter mixture into a small dish for dipping.

Variation: If you like extra kick, grated ginger is a nice addition.

MACRONUTRIENTS	67% FAT	32% PROTEIN	1% CARBS

CALORIES: 514; TOTAL FAT: 38G; PROTEIN: 41G; TOTAL CARBS: 2G; FIBER: 0G; NET CARBS: 2G

MARINATED AND SEARED AHI TUNA

PREP TIME: 5 MINUTES, PLUS OVERNIGHT TO MARINATE **COOK TIME:** 5 MINUTES

What's not to love about a meal you barely have to cook? Seared ahi drizzled with Sriracha mayonnaise is one of my absolute favorite combinations. I like to marinate the tuna steaks overnight to really soak in all the flavor, but you can adjust the marination time to fit your needs. *Serves 2*

○ COMFORT FOOD
◐ DAIRY-FREE
● NUT-FREE
● PALEO OR PALEO-FRIENDLY

2 (8-ounce) fresh ahi tuna steaks

2 tablespoons coconut aminos or soy sauce

1 tablespoon freshly squeezed lemon juice

1 teaspoon garlic powder

1 tablespoon toasted sesame seeds

Salt

Freshly ground black pepper

2 tablespoons cooking oil or ghee

2 tablespoons avocado oil mayonnaise

1 tablespoon Sriracha

1 tablespoon sliced scallions, green parts only

1. Using paper towels, pat the tuna steaks dry and place them in a baking dish.

2. In a small bowl, combine the coconut aminos, lemon juice, garlic powder, and sesame seeds. Season with salt and pepper, and mix well.

3. Pour the marinade over the tuna, coating it on all sides. Cover the dish with plastic wrap and place in the refrigerator. I marinate overnight and turn the steaks once to equally marinate both sides.

4. In a large skillet, heat the cooking oil over high heat. Once the oil is hot, add the tuna steaks and sear each side for 1 to 1½ minutes.

5. Using a spatula, remove the tuna steaks from the skillet and let them rest for 10 minutes.

6. In a small bowl, mix the mayonnaise and Sriracha.

7. Slice the tuna steaks against the grain. Drizzle the Sriracha mayonnaise on top and garnish with the scallions.

| MACRONUTRIENTS | 54% FAT | 43% PROTEIN | 3% CARBS |

CALORIES: 485; TOTAL FAT: 29G; PROTEIN: 52G; TOTAL CARBS: 4G; FIBER: 1G; NET CARBS: 3G

BLACKENED FISH FILLETS
ON SRIRACHA-TOSSED SLAW

PREP TIME: 10 MINUTES **COOK TIME:** 10 MINUTES

Sriracha mayonnaise is one of those sauces that can make almost anything delicious, and this swordfish is no exception. The crunch of the cabbage, the creamy kick of the Sriracha mayonnaise, and the blackened fish is a combination that will make your taste buds super happy! *Serves 2*

○ COMFORT FOOD
◐ DAIRY-FREE
● NUT-FREE
● PALEO OR PALEO-FRIENDLY
○ SUPER QUICK

2 (4- to 6-ounce) swordfish fillets

1 teaspoon paprika

1 teaspoon garlic powder

¼ teaspoon cayenne pepper

Salt

Freshly ground black pepper

1 tablespoon cooking oil or ghee

2 tablespoons avocado oil mayonnaise

1 tablespoon Sriracha

1 cup shredded red cabbage

1. Pat the fish dry with paper towels.

2. In a small bowl, mix the paprika, garlic powder, and cayenne. Season with salt and pepper and mix well.

3. Coat the top and bottom of the fish with the spice mixture.

4. In a medium skillet, add the cooking oil over medium-high heat. Once the pan is hot, add the swordfish fillets. Cook on each side for 3 minutes, until the flesh is slightly blackened on the outside and flakes with a fork.

5. While the fish is cooking, mix the mayonnaise and Sriracha in a small bowl.

6. In a medium bowl, combine the shredded cabbage and half the Sriracha mayonnaise and toss well.

7. Divide the cabbage between two plates and top with the blackened swordfish fillets. Dollop the remaining sriracha mayonnaise on top.

Variation: You can also use sea bass or another firm fish. This is also delicious inside a low-carb tortilla.

MACRONUTRIENTS	61% FAT	34% PROTEIN	5% CARBS

CALORIES: 425; TOTAL FAT: 29G; PROTEIN: 36G; TOTAL CARBS: 5G; FIBER: 2G; NET CARBS: 3G

SPICY MUSSELS

PREP TIME: 15 MINUTES **COOK TIME:** 10 MINUTES

If you've never tried mussels, this recipe is a great way to start! There is a little bit of prep work, but they broil quickly and are easy to make in bulk, which makes them the perfect party appetizer. *Serves 2*

○ COMFORT FOOD
◐ DAIRY-FREE
● NUT-FREE
● PALEO OR PALEO-FRIENDLY
○ SUPER QUICK

12 green mussels, thawed

¼ cup avocado oil mayonnaise

2 tablespoons Sriracha

1 tablespoon coconut aminos or soy sauce

¼ cup ground pork rinds

2 tablespoons sliced scallions, green parts only

1 tablespoon sesame seeds

2 tablespoons masago (smelt roe)

1. Preheat the oven to broil. Line a baking sheet with a silicone mat or parchment paper.

2. Remove the meat from the mussels and cut it into bite-size pieces.

3. In a mixing bowl, combine the mussels, mayonnaise, Sriracha, and coconut aminos. Mix well.

4. Line up the mussel shells on a baking sheet with the open cavity facing up.

5. Divide the mixture between the mussel shells, scooping a spoonful at a time into each.

6. Top with the ground pork rinds and broil for 8 to 10 minutes, until golden brown.

7. Top the mussels with the scallions, sesame seeds, and masago, and serve.

Variation: You can also chop up 5 cooked shrimp and add them to the mussels and sauce mixture.

MACRONUTRIENTS	69% FAT	18% PROTEIN	13% CARBS

CALORIES: 338; TOTAL FAT: 26G; PROTEIN: 15G; TOTAL CARBS: 11G; FIBER: 1G; NET CARBS: 10G

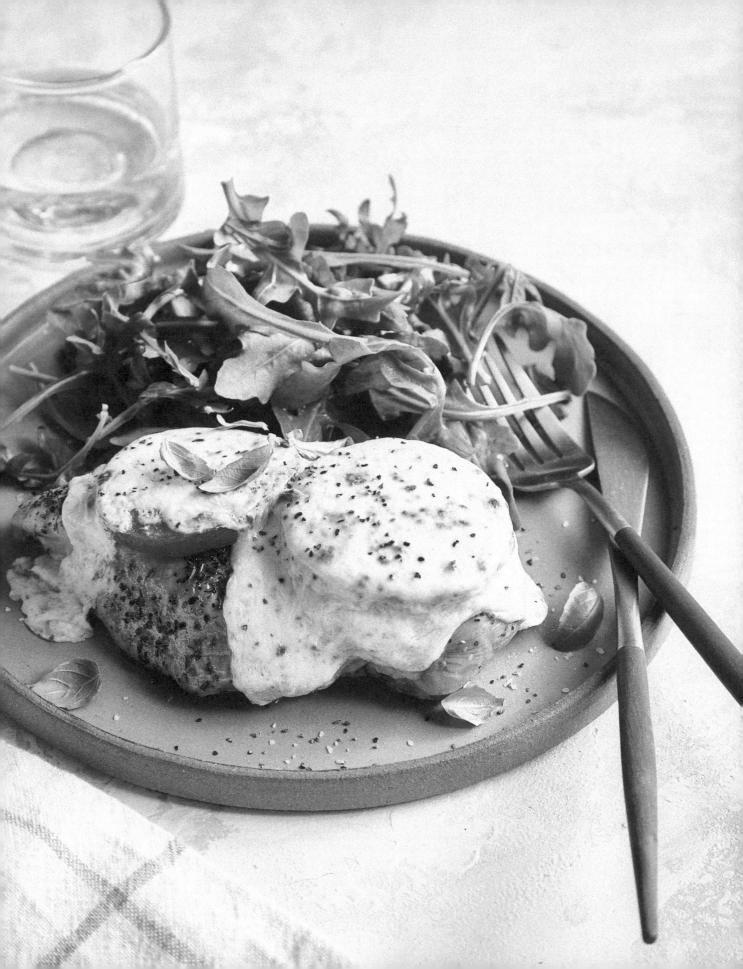

CHICKEN

CHAPTER NINE

Opposite: Caprese Chicken

AVOCADO CHICKEN SALAD

PREP TIME: 10 MINUTES **COOK TIME:** 8 MINUTES

You can use any fresh or leftover baked chicken breast to make this salad, but personally I love the extra flavor that the Shredded Garlic-Lime Chicken (page 153) adds to this salad, so whenever I make that recipe, I end up making this one the next day. *Serves 2*

- ● ALLERGEN-FREE
- ○ COMFORT FOOD
- ◐ DAIRY-FREE
- ● NUT-FREE
- ● PALEO OR PALEO-FRIENDLY
- ○ SUPER QUICK

2 bacon slices

2 tablespoons avocado oil mayonnaise (optional)

1 avocado, halved, pitted and peeled, divided

1 tablespoon freshly squeezed lime juice

Salt

Freshly ground black pepper

1 Shredded Garlic Lime-Chicken breast (page 153)

½ celery stalk, diced

2 tablespoons sliced scallions, green parts only

1. In a large skillet, cook the bacon over medium-high heat for about 8 minutes, flipping once, until crispy. Transfer the bacon to a paper towel–lined plate to drain and cool, then crumble it.

2. In a food processor, add the mayonnaise (if using), half of the avocado, and the lime juice. Season with salt and pepper. Process until smooth.

3. Dice the remaining half of the avocado and put it in a mixing bowl with the chicken, celery, and crumbled bacon.

4. Pour the mixture from the food processor on top and toss to fully combine.

5. Top with the scallions as a garnish and serve.

Variation: Want even more avocado? Scoop the chicken salad into halved avocados as a "bowl." I also like to eat this with butter lettuce cups or romaine leaves for some crunch.

MACRONUTRIENTS	49% FAT	38% PROTEIN	13% CARBS

CALORIES: 308; TOTAL FAT: 17G; PROTEIN: 29G; TOTAL CARBS: 10G; FIBER: 5G; NET CARBS: 5G

SPICY CHICKEN ZOODLE ALFREDO

PREP TIME: 10 MINUTES **COOK TIME:** 15 MINUTES

Who doesn't love some spice in their life? Add a little heat to your Alfredo sauce to kick it up a notch from the standard cream sauce. This dish uses a skillet to cook the chicken while the sauce cooks in a saucepan at the same time, so you'll have dinner in no time. *Serves 2*

○ COMFORT FOOD
● NUT-FREE
○ SUPER QUICK

1 chicken breast

Salt

Freshly ground black pepper

1 tablespoons Italian Seasoning (page 246), plus 1 teaspoon

1 tablespoon extra-virgin olive oil or ghee

4 tablespoons butter

2 ounces cream cheese

½ cup heavy whipping cream

½ cup grated Parmesan cheese

1 garlic clove, finely minced

1 teaspoon Sriracha

½ teaspoon cayenne pepper

2 zucchini, spiralized (zoodles)

1. Pat the chicken breast dry and season both sides with salt, pepper, and 1 tablespoon of Italian seasoning.

2. In a skillet, heat the olive oil over medium heat. Add the chicken and cook for 6 minutes on each side, until the chicken reaches an internal temperature of 165°F and its juices run clear.

3. While the chicken is cooking, in a medium saucepan, combine the butter, cream cheese, and heavy cream over medium heat. Whisk slowly and constantly until the butter and cream cheese melt.

4. Add the Parmesan, garlic, remaining 1 teaspoon of Italian seasoning, Sriracha, and cayenne pepper. Continue to whisk until everything is well blended. Turn the heat to medium-low and simmer, stirring occasionally, for 5 to 8 minutes to allow the sauce to blend and thicken.

5. Remove the cooked chicken from the skillet. Add the zoodles and sauté them in the chicken seasoning for 2 to 3 minutes.

6. Cut the finished chicken into thin slices.

7. Divide the zoodles between two bowls and top with the spicy Alfredo sauce and chicken.

Variation: I also love this dish as a vegetarian dinner when I've eaten too much protein earlier in the day. It's easy to leave out the chicken. Just start cooking at step 3 in the recipe and vary steps 5 and 6 accordingly.

MACRONUTRIENTS (WITHOUT ZOODLES)	88% FAT	10% PROTEIN	2% CARBS

CALORIES: 852; TOTAL FAT: 84G; PROTEIN: 21G; TOTAL CARBS: 5G; FIBER: 0G; NET CARBS: 5G

JALAPEÑO POPPER CHICKEN

PREP TIME: 5 MINUTES **COOK TIME:** 50 MINUTES

One of my favorite keto sides is bacon-wrapped jalapeño peppers stuffed with cream cheese, so it was only natural that I would find a way to sneak this amazing combination into other recipes. The jalapeño seeds are removed in this recipe, so it is kid-friendly as well. *Serves 2*

○ COMFORT FOOD

● NUT-FREE

2 bacon slices

2 boneless skinless chicken breasts

Salt

Freshly ground black pepper

4 ounces cream cheese, at room temperature

3 jalapeño peppers, seeded and sliced

½ cup shredded Mexican blend cheese

1. Preheat the oven to 375°F.

2. In a large skillet, cook the bacon over medium-high heat for about 8 minutes, flipping once, until crispy. Transfer the bacon to a paper towel–lined plate to drain and cool, then crumble it.

3. Pat the chicken dry with a paper towel and season both sides with salt and pepper.

4. In a baking dish, arrange the chicken breasts and spread the cream cheese over the top of the chicken. Layer the jalapeño slices on the chicken breasts, and top with the cheese.

5. Bake for 30 to 40 minutes, or until the chicken reaches an internal temperature of 165°F and its juices run clear.

6. Add the crumbled bacon on top of the casserole and serve.

Make Ahead: This dish reheats very well and can be refrigerated for up to 5 days or frozen for a few months.

MACRONUTRIENTS	62% FAT	35% PROTEIN	3% CARBS

CALORIES: 478; TOTAL FAT: 33G; PROTEIN: 39G; TOTAL CARBS: 4G; FIBER: 1G; NET CARBS: 3G

SLOW COOKER BUFFALO WINGS

PREP TIME: 10 MINUTES **COOK TIME:** 3 HOURS

If I ask my daughter what she wants to eat, she will usually say either sushi or chicken wings. As you can imagine, the wings are much easier to pull off at home than the sushi. I love making these wings in the slow cooker because they get super tender and full of flavor, and then I quickly finish them under the broiler to get that crispy outside. *Serves 2*

○ COMFORT FOOD
◐ DAIRY-FREE
● NUT-FREE
● PALEO OR PALEO-FRIENDLY

2 tablespoons butter or ghee

6 ounces buffalo wing sauce, divided

1 tablespoon Italian Seasoning (page 246)

1 pound chicken wings

Salt

Freshly ground black pepper

1. Preheat the slow cooker on high.

2. In the slow cooker, add the butter, 4 ounces of buffalo wing sauce, and the Italian seasoning. After the butter melts, mix everything until fully combined.

3. Pat the chicken wings dry with a paper towel and season them with salt and pepper. Place the wings in the slow cooker and toss until coated.

4. Cover and cook for 2 hours and 45 minutes.

5. Preheat the broiler.

6. Line a baking sheet with aluminum foil. Place a rack on the prepared baking sheet if you have one. Otherwise, place the wings right on the foil.

7. Brush half the remaining 2 ounces of buffalo wing sauce on the top side of the wings.

8. Cook under the broiler for 2 to 5 minutes, until the wings reach your desired crispiness.

9. Flip the wings, brush the buffalo wing sauce on the other side, and place them back under the broiler for 2 to 5 minutes, or until they reach your desired crispiness.

Variation: I like my wings crispy and on the dry side, but if you like yours saucy, you can heat an additional 2 tablespoons of butter and 4 ounces of wing sauce in a small saucepan on low until melted. Combine them, and then brush the sauce onto the wings once they are out of the broiler.

MACRONUTRIENTS	71% FAT	29% PROTEIN	0% CARBS

CALORIES: 603; TOTAL FAT: 48G; PROTEIN: 42G; TOTAL CARBS: 0G; FIBER: 0G; NET CARBS: 0G

SLOW COOKER PEANUT CHICKEN CURRY
WITH CRISPY CAULIFLOWER RICE

PREP TIME: 5 MINUTES **COOK TIME:** 4 HOURS

I don't make curry dishes all that often, but I have found myself doing it more often since I discovered how easy it is to make a slow cooker version. Generally a dish like this would have potatoes in it, but I find cauliflower rice to be the perfect low-carb companion. *Serves 2*

○ COMFORT FOOD

◑ DAIRY-FREE

● PALEO OR PALEO-FRIENDLY

1 chicken breast, cubed

Salt

Freshly ground black pepper

1 tablespoon curry powder

2 teaspoons ground turmeric

½ teaspoon cayenne pepper

2 cups spinach

2 garlic cloves, minced

½ onion, diced

1 cup chicken broth or chicken bone broth

½ cup full-fat unsweetened coconut milk

¼ cup peanut butter or almond butter

1 batch Cauliflower Rice (page 36)

1. Preheat the slow cooker on high.

2. Pat the chicken dry with a paper towel and season with salt and pepper.

3. In a small bowl, combine the curry powder, turmeric, cayenne pepper, and a pinch of salt.

4. In the slow cooker, combine the chicken, spinach, garlic, and onion, and sprinkle the spice mix on top. Add the chicken broth, coconut milk, and peanut butter.

5. Cover and cook for 4 hours.

6. Divide the cauliflower rice between two plates and spoon the curry over the top.

Variation: Carrots are traditionally used in this dish, but I left them out and substituted with lower-carb spinach. You can easily add bite-size pieces of carrot if you'd like. Kale also works great in this recipe.

MACRONUTRIENTS (WITHOUT CAULIFLOWER RICE)	68% FAT	18% PROTEIN	14% CARBS

CALORIES: 551; TOTAL FAT: 44G; PROTEIN: 24G; TOTAL CARBS: 23G; FIBER: 7G; NET CARBS: 16G

CURRY CHICKEN WITH SHIRATAKI NOODLES

PREP TIME: 5 MINUTES **COOK TIME:** 4 HOURS

This slow cooker red curry dish provides a great pop of flavor. I love eating anything over Shirataki Noodles (page 40) or Zoodles (page 37). This dish is versatile too, because if you add more broth and coconut milk, you can make a soup out of it. *Serves 2*

- ● ALLERGEN-FREE
- ○ COMFORT FOOD
- ◐ DAIRY-FREE
- ● NUT-FREE
- ● PALEO OR PALEO-FRIENDLY

1 chicken breast, cubed

Salt

Freshly ground black pepper

2 garlic cloves, minced

1 tablespoon red curry paste

1 teaspoon ground ginger

1 cup chicken broth or chicken bone broth

½ cup full-fat unsweetened coconut milk

1 batch Shirataki Noodles (page 40) or Zoodles (page 37)

2 tablespoons chopped cilantro

2 lime wedges

1. Preheat the slow cooker on high.

2. Pat the chicken dry with a paper towel and season with salt and pepper.

3. In the slow cooker, combine the chicken, garlic, red curry paste, ground ginger, chicken broth, and coconut milk.

4. Cover and cook for 4 hours.

5. Divide the noodles between two plates and top with the curry and cilantro. Serve the lime wedges on the side.

Variation: As mentioned in the headnote, you can convert this dish into a soup: Just double the amount of chicken broth and coconut milk. You can also add more chicken if you would like more protein.

MACRONUTRIENTS	65% FAT	27% PROTEIN	8% CARBS

CALORIES: 246; TOTAL FAT: 19G; PROTEIN: 16G; TOTAL CARBS: 7G; FIBER: 1G; NET CARBS: 6G

BACON AND BROCCOLI CHICKEN BAKE

PREP TIME: 10 MINUTES **COOK TIME:** 40 MINUTES

I love that you can make this meal in just one dish! Chicken piled with crisp veggies, melted cheese, and salty bacon makes for a delicious combination. *Serves 2*

○ COMFORT FOOD
● NUT-FREE

4 bacon strips

2 boneless chicken breasts

Salt

Freshly ground black pepper

1 cup broccoli florets, fresh or frozen

½ cup shredded Swiss or mozzarella cheese

1. Preheat the oven to 375°F.

2. In a large skillet, cook the bacon over medium-high heat for about 8 minutes, flipping once, until crispy. Transfer the bacon to a paper towel–lined plate to drain and cool, then crumble it.

3. Season the chicken breasts with salt and pepper and transfer to a baking dish.

4. Top the chicken with the broccoli, then the bacon, then the cheese.

5. Bake uncovered for 30 to 40 minutes, or until the chicken reaches an internal temperature of 165°F and the cheese is browned and golden.

Variation: Bell peppers also work nicely if you don't have broccoli on hand.

MACRONUTRIENTS	57% FAT	40% PROTEIN	3% CARBS

CALORIES: 406; TOTAL FAT: 26G; PROTEIN: 39G; TOTAL CARBS: 3G; FIBER: 1G; NET CARBS: 2G

CAPRESE CHICKEN

PREP TIME: 5 MINUTES **COOK TIME:** 40 MINUTES

Caprese is proof that the most delicious things can also be very simple. This dish tops chicken breasts with gooey mozzarella, Roma tomatoes, and fresh basil. *Serves 2*

○ COMFORT FOOD
● NUT-FREE

2 chicken breasts

1 tablespoon Italian Seasoning (page 246)

Salt

Freshly ground black pepper

4 (½-inch-thick) slices Roma tomato

4 (1-ounce) slices mozzarella cheese

2 tablespoons chopped fresh basil

1. Preheat the oven to 375°F.

2. Pat the chicken dry with a paper towel and season both sides with Italian seasoning, salt, and pepper.

3. In a baking dish, arrange the chicken breasts and top each breast with 2 tomato slices and then 2 slices of mozzarella.

4. Bake for 30 to 40 minutes, or until the chicken reaches an internal temperature of 165°F and the juices run clear.

5. Garnish with the basil and serve.

Variation: You can add 2 tablespoons of pesto for even more flavor. I use a prepared pesto and just slather it on both chicken breasts before topping with the tomato, cheese, and basil. I also like to pair this rich, cheesy chicken with arugula, which adds a kick of freshness.

MACRONUTRIENTS	56% FAT	42% PROTEIN	2% CARBS

CALORIES: 367; TOTAL FAT: 23G; PROTEIN: 36G; TOTAL CARBS: 3G; FIBER: 0G; NET CARBS: 3G

PORK RIND—CRUSTED CHICKEN TENDERS

PREP TIME: 15 MINUTES **COOK TIME:** 10 MINUTES

No need to miss breaded chicken tenders—these are even better! These tenders are super crispy and easy to make, and you'll be dipping them in no time. *Serves 2*

○ COMFORT FOOD
◐ DAIRY-FREE
● PALEO OR PALEO-FRIENDLY
○ SUPER QUICK

1 large egg

½ cup coconut flour

1 teaspoon cayenne pepper

Salt

Freshly ground black pepper

1 batch Pork Rind "Bread" Crumbs (page 249)

2 tablespoons extra-virgin olive oil or ghee

1 pound boneless, skinless chicken tenders (about 8 tenders)

1. In a shallow bowl, lightly beat the egg. On a large plate, mix the coconut flour and cayenne pepper. Season with salt and pepper. On another large plate, put the pork rind "bread" crumbs.

2. In a large skillet, heat the olive oil over medium-high heat.

3. Dredge each tender on both sides in the coconut flour mixture. Dip the tender into the egg, coating on both sides. Dredge in the pork rind crumbs, pressing the pork rinds into the chicken so they stick. Place the coated chicken tender into the hot skillet. Repeat with the remaining chicken tenders.

4. Cook each tender for 3 minutes on each side, until it is brown, crispy, and cooked through.

Variation: This combination makes an excellent base for all kinds of flavoring options. Add other seasonings to the coconut flour mixture, including the seasoning mixes in chapter 14.

MACRONUTRIENTS	39% FAT	48% PROTEIN	13% CARBS

CALORIES: 550; TOTAL FAT: 24G; PROTEIN: 63G; TOTAL CARBS: 17G; FIBER: 11G; NET CARBS: 6G

CHICKEN-FRIED CAULIFLOWER RICE CASSEROLE

PREP TIME: 10 MINUTES **COOK TIME:** 30 MINUTES

Miss fried rice on the keto diet? Look no further! This version is a casserole, which I love because you can throw it in the oven and do something else while it cooks, and as a single mom, I am ALWAYS multitasking! *Serves 2*

○ COMFORT FOOD
◐ DAIRY-FREE
● NUT-FREE
● PALEO OR PALEO-FRIENDLY

1 chicken breast, cubed

Salt

Freshly ground black pepper

1 tablespoon sesame oil

½ bell pepper, diced

½ cauliflower head, riced

1 garlic clove, pressed

1 teaspoon ground ginger

1 teaspoon onion powder

1 teaspoon fish sauce

2 tablespoons soy sauce or coconut aminos

2 large eggs, lightly beaten

2 tablespoons sliced scallions

1. Preheat the oven to 375°F.

2. Pat the chicken dry with a paper towel and season with salt and pepper.

3. In a skillet, heat the sesame oil over medium-high heat. Add the chicken and sauté for about 8 minutes, flipping once, until it is cooked through.

4. Add the bell pepper, cauliflower rice, garlic, ginger, onion powder, fish sauce, and soy sauce to the chicken and sauté for about 5 minutes.

5. Put the entire mixture in a baking dish, then pour the eggs over the top.

6. Bake for 15 minutes.

7. Serve garnished with the scallions.

Make Ahead: This is a great dish to make a double batch of and heat up throughout the week.

MACRONUTRIENTS	56% FAT	32% PROTEIN	12% CARBS

CALORIES: 276; TOTAL FAT: 17G; PROTEIN: 22G; TOTAL CARBS: 9G; FIBER: 3G; NET CARBS: 6G

CREAMY LEMON-GARLIC CHICKEN THIGHS

PREP TIME: 10 MINUTES **COOK TIME:** 40 MINUTES

I grew up in the kind of family that ate only boneless, skinless chicken breast. I don't remember my mom making any other kind of chicken, and because of it, I had an aversion to chicken for a long time. I never bought bone-in chicken thighs until a few years ago. I'm glad I finally did, though, because the dark meat and crispy skin are amazing! This recipe uses an oven-safe skillet, but if you don't have one, just transfer the chicken and sauce to a baking dish before putting it in the oven. *Serves 2*

○ COMFORT FOOD
● NUT-FREE

3 tablespoons extra-virgin olive oil or ghee, divided

2 bone-in chicken thighs, skin on

Salt

Freshly ground black pepper

1 teaspoon Italian Seasoning (page 246)

1 tablespoon cayenne pepper

2 garlic cloves, minced

½ cup heavy whipping cream

¼ cup chicken broth or chicken bone broth

½ cup grated Parmesan cheese

½ lemon, juiced

1 teaspoon dried parsley

1. Preheat the oven to 375°F.

2. In an oven-safe skillet, heat 2 tablespoons of olive oil over medium-high heat.

3. Pat the chicken thighs dry with a paper towel and season both sides with salt, pepper, Italian seasoning, and cayenne pepper. Cook for 3 minutes per side, until the skin is crispy and golden.

4. Remove the chicken from the skillet and set aside on a plate. If necessary, drain any extra fat from the skillet.

5. In the skillet, add the remaining 1 tablespoon of olive oil and garlic and sauté for 1 minute.

6. Stir in the heavy cream, chicken broth, Parmesan cheese, lemon juice, and dried parsley. Let the sauce just barely boil and reduce the heat to low. Simmer for 3 minutes.

7. Add the chicken back into the sauce and place the skillet in oven for 30 minutes, until the chicken reaches an internal temperature of 165°F and its juices run clear.

Variation: This pairs nicely with Roasted Garlic Broccoli with Almonds (page 212), but you can also use the sauce as a pasta sauce with Zoodles (page 37) or Shirataki Noodles (page 40).

MACRONUTRIENTS	81% FAT	15% PROTEIN	4% CARBS

CALORIES: 640; TOTAL FAT: 59G; PROTEIN: 22G; TOTAL CARBS: 8G; FIBER: 1G; NET CARBS: 7G

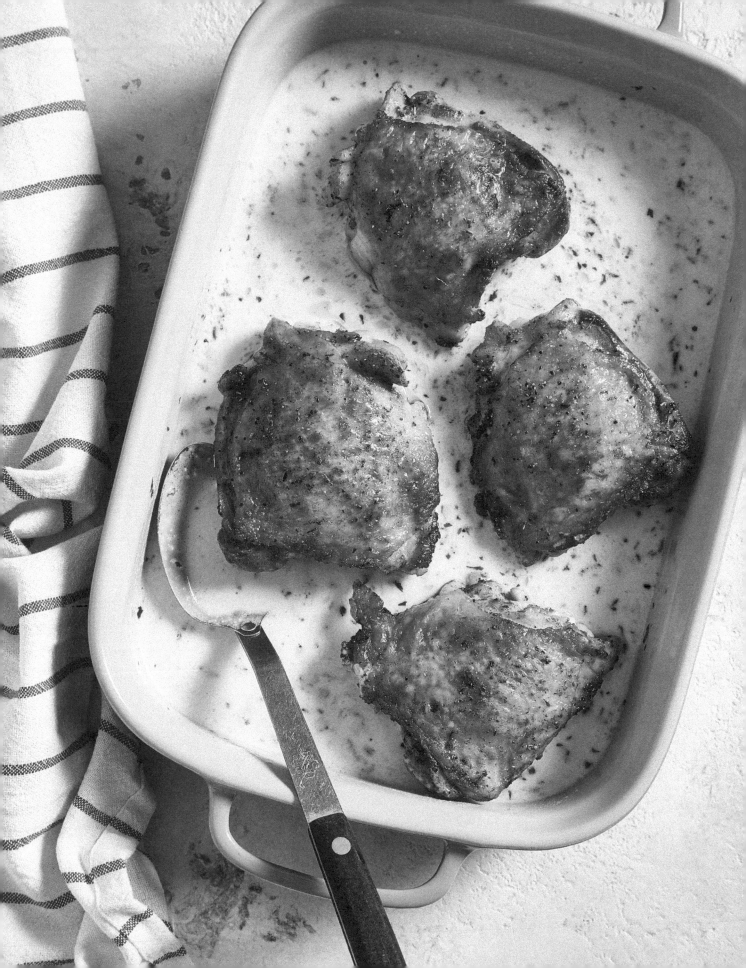

BAKED DIJON CHICKEN LEGS

PREP TIME: 10 MINUTES **COOK TIME:** 50 MINUTES

I love adding Dijon mustard to recipes—it takes everything to the next level, and these are no exception. Making drumsticks is great because they are inexpensive, and they are also my daughter's favorite cut of chicken. If you like yours crispy, don't skip the broiler step! *Serves 2*

● ALLERGEN-FREE
○ COMFORT FOOD
◐ DAIRY-FREE
● NUT-FREE
● PALEO OR PALEO-FRIENDLY

1 pound chicken drumsticks

Salt

Freshly ground black pepper

2 tablespoons extra-virgin olive oil

1 garlic clove, minced

½ teaspoon paprika

1 teaspoon Italian Seasoning (page 246)

1 tablespoon dried parsley

2 tablespoons Dijon mustard

1 tablespoon freshly squeezed lemon juice

1. Preheat the oven to 425°F. Line a baking sheet with aluminum foil or a silicone baking mat.

2. Pat the chicken dry with a paper towel and transfer to a large bowl. Season with salt and pepper.

3. In a small bowl, put the olive oil, garlic, paprika, Italian seasoning, parsley, Dijon, and lemon juice. Whisk to combine and pour over the drumsticks.

4. Marinate the chicken while the oven heats up, and when it's ready, arrange the chicken on the prepared baking sheet.

5. Bake for 50 minutes, flipping the chicken once halfway through. If you want the skin extra crispy, you can turn on the broiler for the last few minutes.

6. Brush the cooked chicken legs with extra sauce from the baking sheet and serve.

Make Ahead: Chicken legs are my daughter's favorite after-school snack, so if your family is like mine, I recommend making extra. I guarantee they will be eaten! You can also marinate this chicken overnight if you want it to soak in extra flavor.

MACRONUTRIENTS	67% FAT	30% PROTEIN	3% CARBS

CALORIES: 316; TOTAL FAT: 24G; PROTEIN: 23G; TOTAL CARBS: 2G; FIBER: 1G; NET CARBS: 1G

DAIRY-FREE CHICKEN ALFREDO WITH MUSHROOMS

PREP TIME: 5 MINUTES **COOK TIME:** 15 MINUTES

I eat full-fat dairy, but I dabble at times with going dairy-free, and this was one of my first recipes in that direction. I figured if I could make a decadent Alfredo sauce without dairy, then everything else would be a piece of cake. Turns out it is super easy! *Serves 2*

○ COMFORT FOOD
◐ DAIRY-FREE
● NUT-FREE
● PALEO OR PALEO-FRIENDLY
○ SUPER QUICK

1 chicken breast

1 tablespoon Italian Seasoning (page 246)

Salt

Freshly ground black pepper

1 tablespoon extra-virgin olive oil

2 tablespoons ghee

½ onion, diced

2 garlic cloves, minced

8 ounces mushrooms, sliced

1 tablespoon coconut flour

7 ounces unsweetened full-fat coconut milk

2 zucchini, spiralized (zoodles)

1. Pat the chicken dry and season both sides with the Italian seasoning, salt, and pepper.

2. In a small skillet, heat the olive oil over medium heat. Cook the chicken for about 6 minutes on each side, until the chicken reaches an internal temperature of 165°F and its juices run clear.

3. While the chicken is cooking, in a medium saucepan, heat the ghee over medium heat. Cook the onion, garlic, and mushrooms, sautéing for about 5 minutes while stirring occasionally, until the vegetables soften.

4. Whisk in the coconut flour and add the coconut milk, whisking until smooth.

5. Bring the sauce to a simmer, whisking occasionally for about 5 minutes, until the sauce thickens. Season with salt.

6. Remove the cooked chicken from the skillet. Add the zoodles to the skillet and sauté them in the chicken seasoning for 2 to 3 minutes.

7. Cut the chicken into thin slices.

8. Divide the zoodles into two bowls and top with the Alfredo sauce and then the sliced chicken.

Variation: You can substitute other vegetables for the mushrooms if desired. Asparagus, broccoli, and cauliflower would all be delicious!

MACRONUTRIENTS	70% FAT	19% PROTEIN	11% CARBS

CALORIES: 464; TOTAL FAT: 36G; PROTEIN: 22G; TOTAL CARBS: 13G; FIBER: 3G; NET CARBS: 10G

SLOW COOKER CHICKEN ENCHILADA BOWLS

PREP TIME: 5 MINUTES **COOK TIME:** 8 HOURS

Chicken enchiladas were my go-to order at Mexican restaurants pre-keto, but I don't even miss them after creating this delicious bowl of goodness. The chicken cooks all day in the homemade enchilada sauce and tastes incredible. Why homemade sauce? Most enchilada sauces are not gluten-free, but if you find a clean one, by all means use it! You can add Cauliflower Rice (page 36) to this recipe, but it's filling without it, so I generally don't. *Serves 2*

○ COMFORT FOOD

● NUT-FREE

2 chicken breasts

¼ cup Enchilada Sauce (page 252)

½ onion, diced

2 ounces canned diced green chiles

¼ cup shredded Mexican blend cheese

1 avocado, pitted, peeled, and diced

1 jalapeño pepper, sliced (optional)

2 tablespoons sour cream

1 teaspoon Chili-Lime Seasoning (page 244) (optional)

1. Preheat the slow cooker on low.

2. In the slow cooker, add the chicken, enchilada sauce, onion, and green chiles.

3. Cover and cook for 8 hours.

4. When the cooking is complete, using two forks, shred the chicken and mix it back into the sauce.

5. Divide the chicken and sauce between two bowls.

6. Top with the shredded cheese, avocado, jalapeño (if using), and sour cream. Sprinkle a little chili-lime seasoning (if using) on top of the sour cream and serve.

Make It Paleo: Use the Dairy-Free Sour Cream (page 259) and leave off the shredded cheese or use a dairy-free alternative.

MACRONUTRIENTS	60% FAT	28% PROTEIN	12% CARBS

CALORIES: 427; TOTAL FAT: 28G; PROTEIN: 30G; TOTAL CARBS: 13G; FIBER: 7G; NET CARBS: 6G

SHREDDED GARLIC-LIME CHICKEN

PREP TIME: 5 MINUTES **COOK TIME:** 8 HOURS

Letting chicken cook low and slow is my favorite way to prepare it. I use shredded chicken in all kinds of recipes, like the Avocado Chicken Salad (page 138), low-carb quesadillas, and pork rind nachos. There are so many options! I used to use store-bought rotisserie chickens, which is easy, but this packs way more flavor. Just know that the chicken alone doesn't really offer much fat, but whatever you top it with can. *Serves 2*

● ALLERGEN-FREE
○ COMFORT FOOD
◔ DAIRY-FREE
● NUT-FREE
● PALEO OR PALEO-FRIENDLY

2 chicken breasts

½ onion, diced

2 garlic cloves, minced

½ lime, zested and juiced

1 teaspoon Chili-Lime Seasoning (page 244)

1 cup chicken broth or chicken bone broth

1 jalapeño pepper, diced

Salt

Freshly ground black pepper

1. Preheat the slow cooker on low.

2. In the slow cooker, combine the chicken, onion, garlic, lime juice and zest, chili-lime seasoning, chicken broth, and jalapeño pepper. Season with salt and pepper.

3. Cover and cook for 8 hours.

4. When the cooking is complete, using two forks, shred both breasts and mix the chicken back into the sauce.

Variation: This chicken is high in flavor on its own, but it is meant to be used in other recipes where you add fats, like avocado, which will keep you satiated.

MACRONUTRIENTS	44% FAT	48% PROTEIN	8% CARBS

CALORIES: 229; TOTAL FAT: 11G; PROTEIN: 26G; TOTAL CARBS: 5G; FIBER: 1G; NET CARBS: 4G

CHICKEN CHEESE CHIP NACHOS

PREP TIME: 10 MINUTES **COOK TIME:** 15 MINUTES

There are lots of fun ways to make keto-friendly nachos. I make pork rind nachos all the time, and I also LOVE the Cheeseless Roasted Cauliflower Nachos (page 232), but this version of nachos is awesome because each chip has ALL the toppings. There is no bad bite! *Serves 2*

○ COMFORT FOOD
● NUT-FREE
○ SUPER QUICK

1 cup shredded Mexican blend cheese

1 tablespoon Taco Seasoning (page 245)

1 tablespoon sour cream

1 avocado

1 tablespoon freshly squeezed lime juice

Cilantro, for garnish

Salt

Freshly ground black pepper

½ cup Shredded Garlic-Lime Chicken (page 153)

1. Preheat the oven to 350°F. Line a baking sheet with parchment paper or a silicone baking mat.

2. Add ¼-cup mounds of shredded cheese to the pan, leaving plenty of space between them, and sprinkle each cheese mound with the taco seasoning.

3. Bake for about 7 minutes, until the edges are brown and the middles have fully melted.

4. Set the pan on a cooling rack, and let the cheese chips cool for 5 minutes. The chips will be floppy when they first come out of the oven but will crisp as they cool, so don't move them for 5 minutes.

5. While the cheese chips are cooling, in a food processor or blender, combine the sour cream, avocado, lime juice, and cilantro. Season with salt and pepper. Process until smooth and fully combined.

6. Top the cheese chips with the shredded chicken and avocado crema. Garnish with a bit more cilantro and serve.

Variation: In my first cookbook, I have a recipe for Avocado-Lime Crema. I used a simpler version without garlic in this recipe because the Garlic-Lime Chicken is so full of flavor, but feel free to use it and double up on flavor if you want!

MACRONUTRIENTS	68% FAT	28% PROTEIN	4% CARBS

CALORIES: 354; TOTAL FAT: 27G; PROTEIN: 26G; TOTAL CARBS: 5G; FIBER: 1G; NET CARBS: 4G

MEXICAN CAULIFLOWER RICE
WITH SHREDDED CHICKEN

PREP TIME: 10 MINUTES **COOK TIME:** 8 HOURS 15 MINUTES

This dish is like a Mexican take on fried rice. Yum! I use cauliflower rice and spice it up with bell peppers, jalapeño peppers, and taco seasoning, and then top it off with the same flavorful chicken from the Slow Cooker Chicken Enchilada Bowls (page 152). The result is delicious, and if you already have the chicken made, this will take you less than 15 minutes. I use only about 1 cup of the shredded chicken (½ cup per person) for this recipe, so I have some leftovers. *Serves 2*

● ALLERGEN-FREE
○ COMFORT FOOD
◐ DAIRY-FREE
● NUT-FREE
● PALEO OR PALEO-FRIENDLY

*FOR THE SLOW COOKER
ENCHILADA CHICKEN*

2 chicken breasts

¼ cup Enchilada Sauce (page 252)

½ onion, diced

2 ounces canned diced green chiles

TO MAKE THE SLOW COOKER ENCHILADA CHICKEN

1. Preheat the slow cooker on low.

2. In the slow cooker, add the chicken, enchilada sauce, onion, and green chiles.

3. Cover and cook for 8 hours.

4. Remove the chicken and shred, using two forks, and mix back into the sauce.

continued

MACRONUTRIENTS	53% FAT	29% PROTEIN	18% CARBS

CALORIES: 388; TOTAL FAT: 23G; PROTEIN: 28G; TOTAL CARBS: 18G; FIBER: 7G; NET CARBS: 11G

FOR THE MEXICAN CAULIFLOWER RICE

1 tablespoon extra-virgin olive oil

½ onion, diced

1 garlic clove, minced

1 jalapeño pepper, diced

½ Roma tomato, diced

¼ cup diced red, green, or yellow bell peppers

2 teaspoons Taco Seasoning (page 245)

½ cauliflower head, riced

Salt

Freshly ground black pepper

½ avocado, diced

TO MAKE THE MEXICAN CAULIFLOWER RICE

1. In a large skillet, heat the olive oil over medium-high heat.

2. Add the onion, garlic, and jalapeño pepper and cook until softened, about 5 minutes.

3. Add the tomato, bell pepper, and taco seasoning to the skillet. Stir to combine all the ingredients.

4. Add the cauliflower rice to the skillet and season with salt and pepper. Cook for 5 minutes, stirring frequently, or if you like it a little crispy like I do, for 10 minutes.

5. Divide between two bowls and top with the enchilada chicken and diced avocado.

Variation: Dairy-Free Sour Cream (page 259) or Dairy-Free Avocado Crema (page 257) would also make great toppings.

BACON-WRAPPED CREAM CHEESE CHICKEN

PREP TIME: 10 MINUTES **COOK TIME:** 50 MINUTES

Wrap pretty much anything in bacon and I will be excited to eat it! I decided to make this with my Dairy-Free Cream Cheese (page 258), but you can use regular cream cheese instead. You can also add any number of seasonings to the cream cheese to customize this. *Serves 2*

○ COMFORT FOOD

◐ DAIRY-FREE

● PALEO OR PALEO-FRIENDLY

6 bacon slices

2 chicken breasts

Salt

Freshly ground black pepper

4 ounces Dairy-Free Cream Cheese (page 258) or cream cheese, at room temperature

1. Preheat the oven to 375°F.

2. In a large skillet over medium-high heat, cook the bacon until it's around halfway done, about 4 minutes. You want it floppy and pliable. Transfer to a plate.

3. While the bacon is cooking, pound the chicken breasts with a mallet (if you don't have one, a heavy plate, rolling pin, or wine bottle will do the trick). You want the chicken about ½ inch thick so it is easy to roll.

4. Pat the chicken dry with a paper towel and season both sides with salt and pepper.

5. Spread the softened cream cheese into the middle of the inside of the pounded chicken breasts. Then roll the chicken from the short side into a log-like shape so that the cream cheese is inside.

6. Wrap 3 pieces of the bacon around each chicken breast and place them in the baking dish with the seam side down. You can use toothpicks to keep the bacon in place.

7. Bake for 40 minutes, or until the bacon is crispy.

Variation: The cream cheese is a blank palate for flavors. I like to add chopped pepperoncini to mine. Mix it into the cream cheese and spread—or just sprinkle it on top before rolling the chicken up.

MACRONUTRIENTS	69% FAT	29% PROTEIN	2% CARBS

CALORIES: 514; TOTAL FAT: 40G; PROTEIN: 36G; TOTAL CARBS: 3G; FIBER: 0G; NET CARBS: 3G

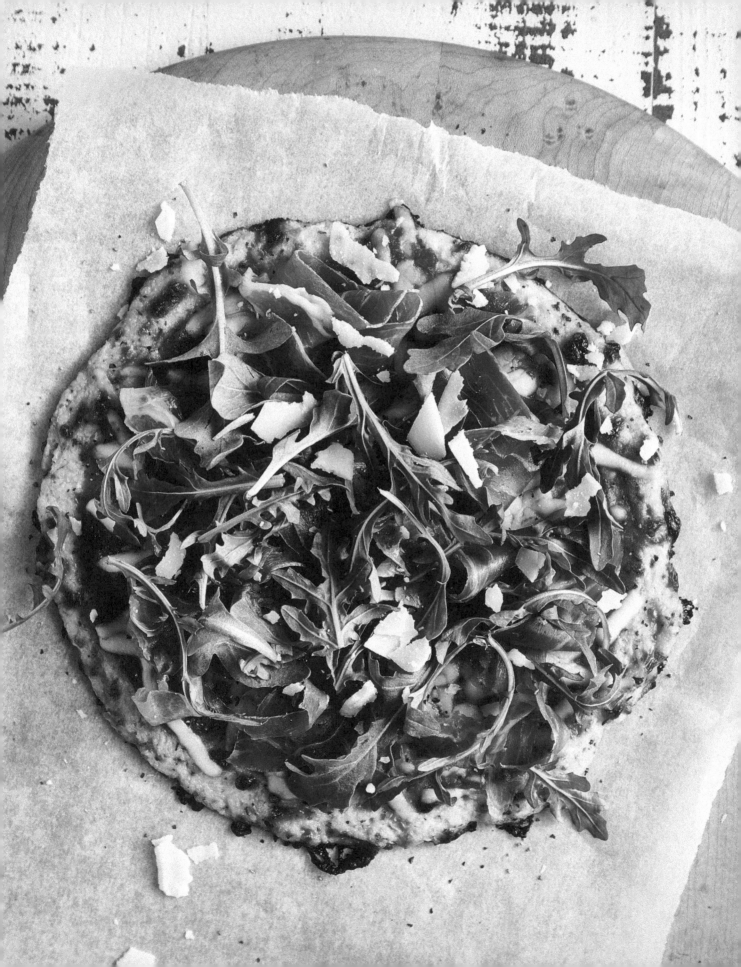

PORK

CHAPTER TEN

Opposite: Prosciutto and Arugula Cauliflower Crust Pizza

MOZZARELLA PROSCIUTTO BOMBS

PREP TIME: 5 MINUTES **COOK TIME:** 10 MINUTES

Imagine a cheese bomb wrapped in crispy prosciutto with fresh pops of basil and tomato. Sounds amazing, right? These make great appetizers or a creative meal. I make them with the tiny marinated mozzarella balls, but they work just as well with larger chunks. *Serves 2*

○ COMFORT FOOD
● NUT-FREE
○ SUPER QUICK

6 small mozzarella balls (I use the marinated variety)

12 prosciutto slices

6 grape tomatoes

6 fresh basil leaves

1 teaspoon Italian Seasoning (page 246)

2 tablespoons extra-virgin olive oil

1. On a work surface, make a cross with 2 slices of prosciutto.

2. Using a knife, hollow out a hole in the middle of a mozzarella ball and stuff a grape tomato inside.

3. Place a basil leaf and a tomato-stuffed mozzarella ball in the middle of the crossed prosciutto slices and add a pinch Italian seasoning.

4. Cross the left and then the right prosciutto slice over the mozzarella ball. Then cross the upper and lower prosciutto slices over that. Repeat with the remaining mozzarella balls.

5. In a skillet over medium-high heat, heat the olive oil. Once hot, add the mozzarella prosciutto bombs and cook on the top and bottom, until crispy. Quickly sear the sides at the end of cooking.

6. Transfer to a paper towel–lined plate to cool and serve.

Make Ahead: These reheat really well if you want to make extra.

MACRONUTRIENTS	70% FAT	28% PROTEIN	2% CARBS

CALORIES: 450; TOTAL FAT: 35G; PROTEIN: 31G; TOTAL CARBS: 2G; FIBER: 1G; NET CARBS: 1G

PROSCIUTTO-WRAPPED PEPPERS

PREP TIME: 10 MINUTES **COOK TIME:** 15 MINUTES

This is a lighter meal that is perfect when you just want a small plate. It reminds me of tapas restaurants where you order lots of small plates, which I love. These are a perfectly grown-up version of a standard popper. *Serves 2*

○ COMFORT FOOD
● NUT-FREE
○ SUPER QUICK

½ jalapeño pepper, diced

2 ounces cream cheese or Dairy-Free Cream Cheese (page 258)

¼ cup artichoke hearts, drained and chopped

1 teaspoon garlic powder

2 bell peppers, cut into quarters

4 prosciutto slices, halved lengthwise, plus more as needed

1. Preheat the oven to 450°F. Line a baking sheet with parchment paper or a silicone baking mat.

2. In a small bowl, mix the jalapeño pepper, cream cheese, artichoke hearts, and garlic powder.

3. Spoon the mixture into the bell peppers and then wrap the peppers with prosciutto. Use half a slice cut lengthwise for each pepper. If your peppers are larger, you may need to use a little more prosciutto.

4. Bake for 12 minutes. Turn on the broiler and broil for 1 additional minute, until crispy.

Variation: You can add additional diced veggies or herbs to the mixture if you want. Parmesan cheese is also a nice addition.

MACRONUTRIENTS	61% FAT	20% PROTEIN	19% CARBS

CALORIES: 236; TOTAL FAT: 16G; PROTEIN: 12G; TOTAL CARBS: 11G; FIBER: 2G; NET CARBS: 9G

PEPPERONI AND PEPPERONCINI FATHEAD PIZZA

PREP TIME: 20 MINUTES **COOK TIME:** 20 MINUTES

Don't be intimidated by the long list of ingredients. FatHead pizza is easy to make and tastes just like the carb-filled kind of pizza! You can get creative with your toppings, but pepperoni and pepperoncini, or green olives, are my favorites. *Serves 4*

○ **COMFORT FOOD**

FOR THE FATHEAD DOUGH

1¾ cups shredded mozzarella cheese

2 tablespoons cream cheese or Dairy-Free Cream Cheese (page 258)

¾ cup almond flour

1 large egg

1 teaspoon Italian Seasoning (page 246)

Pinch salt

Nonstick cooking spray

TO MAKE THE FATHEAD DOUGH

1. Preheat the oven to 425°F.

2. In a microwave-safe bowl, combine the shredded cheese and cream cheese, and microwave on high for 1 minute. Stir the mixture and microwave again for 30 more seconds, until melted.

3. Add the almond flour, egg, Italian seasoning, and salt to the cheese mixture and mix everything together gently.

4. Lightly spray two pieces of parchment paper with cooking spray and place the dough ball between the pieces. Using a rolling pin (or wine bottle in a pinch!), roll the dough into the desired shape.

5. Peel off the top piece of parchment paper and place the dough and bottom piece of parchment onto a baking sheet.

6. Form a crust by pinching or rolling the edges and then, using a fork, poke about 20 holes all over the dough.

7. Bake for 12 to 15 minutes, until the dough is golden brown.

MACRONUTRIENTS	71% FAT	25% PROTEIN	4% CARBS

CALORIES: 416; TOTAL FAT: 33G; PROTEIN: 25G; TOTAL CARBS: 5G; FIBER: 1G; NET CARBS: 4G

½ cup sugar-free tomato sauce

½ cup shredded mozzarella cheese

¼ cup grated Parmesan cheese

3 ounces pepperoni

3 ounces sliced pepperoncini
or olives

2 tablespoons thinly sliced
fresh basil

1. Add the tomato sauce to the crust and spread evenly.

2. Add the mozzarella cheese, Parmesan cheese, pepperoni, and pepperoncini.

3. Bake for 5 minutes, until the cheese melts.

4. Top with the basil and serve.

Variation: Sometimes I use chunks of diced tomatoes instead of tomato sauce.

SPICY SLOW COOKER SHREDDED PORK

PREP TIME: 5 MINUTES **COOK TIME:** 8 HOURS

Shredded pork is a constant in my household. It's delicious by itself or when added to other dishes like pork rind nachos or low-carb quesadillas. You can crank up the seasoning if you like spicy food. *Serves 2*

- ● ALLERGEN-FREE
- ○ COMFORT FOOD
- ◐ DAIRY-FREE
- ● NUT-FREE
- ● PALEO OR PALEO-FRIENDLY

1 (1-pound) pork butt roast

Salt

Freshly ground black pepper

1 tablespoon dried oregano

1 tablespoon ground cumin

½ small onion, diced

2 garlic cloves, minced

1 jalapeño pepper, chopped

½ lime, juiced

1. Season the pork with salt and pepper, and the oregano and cumin.

2. In the slow cooker, add the pork and top it with the onion, garlic, jalapeño, and lime juice.

3. Cover and cook on low for 8 hours.

4. Shred the meat with two forks and serve.

Make Ahead: To reheat the pork, I recommend adding the meat and some juices to a hot skillet and heating until the edges are a little crispy.

MACRONUTRIENTS	57% FAT	39% PROTEIN	4% CARBS

CALORIES: 412; TOTAL FAT: 26G; PROTEIN: 40G; TOTAL CARBS: 6G; FIBER: 2G; NET CARBS: 4G

PROSCIUTTO AND ARUGULA CAULIFLOWER CRUST PIZZA

PREP TIME: 15 MINUTES **COOK TIME:** 25 MINUTES

The Pepperoni and Pepperoncini FatHead Pizza (page 162) is a great keto pizza option, but this cauliflower crust is also a delicious way to keto-fy one of the world's ultimate comfort foods. You bake the crust first and then top as you wish. I love the tangy combination of salty prosciutto and fresh arugula. *Serves 2*

○ COMFORT FOOD
● NUT-FREE

½ cauliflower head, broken into florets

1 large egg, beaten

1 cup shredded mozzarella cheese, divided

2 tablespoons grated Parmesan cheese

1 teaspoon Italian Seasoning (page 246)

1 tablespoon extra-virgin olive oil, divided

2 tablespoons low-sugar marinara sauce

2 cups arugula

Salt

Freshly ground black pepper

4 prosciutto slices, torn into smaller pieces

1 tablespoon shaved Parmesan cheese

1. Preheat the oven to 425°F. Line a baking sheet with parchment paper or a silicone baking mat.

2. Place the cauliflower in the food processor and pulse until finely ground.

3. In a microwave-safe bowl, cook the cauliflower for 4 to 5 minutes, until soft. Transfer to a clean kitchen towel and cool. Once it is cooled, squeeze the towel and wring out as much moisture as possible.

4. In a bowl, mix the cauliflower, egg, ½ cup of mozzarella, the grated Parmesan, and the Italian seasoning. Mix well and transfer the dough to the baking sheet. Form it into a ½-inch-thick circle (or desired shape) and bake for 15 minutes, until golden.

5. Brush the crust with ½ tablespoon of olive oil. Top with the marinara sauce and the remaining ½ cup of mozzarella cheese. Bake for 5 minutes, until the cheese is melted and bubbling.

6. Meanwhile, toss the arugula with the remaining ½ tablespoon of olive oil and season with salt and pepper.

7. Remove the pizza from the oven and top with the arugula, prosciutto, and shaved Parmesan.

MACRONUTRIENTS	63% FAT	30% PROTEIN	7% CARBS

CALORIES: 344; TOTAL FAT: 24G; PROTEIN: 26G; TOTAL CARBS: 6G; FIBER: 2G; NET CARBS: 4G

GROUND PORK EGG ROLL SLAW

PREP TIME: 5 MINUTES **COOK TIME:** 20 MINUTES

This is one of the most popular keto-friendly recipes, as it has all the flavors of an egg roll, but in a keto-friendly bowl. Be warned that this dish can be super addicting, and you might just find yourself eating it every day. *Serves 2*

○ COMFORT FOOD
◐ DAIRY-FREE
● NUT-FREE
● PALEO OR PALEO-FRIENDLY
○ SUPER QUICK

1 tablespoon sesame oil

2 garlic cloves, minced

¼ onion, diced

½ pound ground pork

2 teaspoons Sriracha

Salt

Freshly ground black pepper

1 tablespoon soy sauce or coconut aminos

2 teaspoons rice wine vinegar

2 cups coleslaw mix

¼ cup sliced scallions, green parts only

1 tablespoon sesame seeds

1. In a skillet, heat the sesame oil over medium-high heat. Add the garlic and onion and cook for 1 to 2 minutes, until softened.

2. Add the ground pork and Sriracha, and season with salt and pepper. Cook for 8 to 10 minutes, breaking up the pork and stirring occasionally.

3. Add the soy sauce and vinegar and stir well.

4. Add the coleslaw mix to the skillet and sauté for 3 to 5 minutes, until the cabbage softens.

5. Divide between two bowls, and top with the scallions and sesame seeds.

Variation: You can easily substitute ground beef or chicken for the ground pork.

MACRONUTRIENTS	70% FAT	22% PROTEIN	8% CARBS

CALORIES: 423; TOTAL FAT: 33G; PROTEIN: 22G; TOTAL CARBS: 10G; FIBER: 3G; NET CARBS: 7G

BACON-WRAPPED PORK NUGGETS

PREP TIME: 10 MINUTES **COOK TIME:** 15 MINUTES

Pork wrapped in more pork? Yes, please! Who needs chicken nuggets when you can make these? I love bacon around pretty much anything, and boneless pork chops are often super affordable, making this a satisfying and budget-friendly dish. Plus, kids will love them. *Serves 2*

● ALLERGEN-FREE
○ COMFORT FOOD
◐ DAIRY-FREE
● NUT-FREE
● PALEO OR PALEO-FRIENDLY
○ SUPER QUICK

8 bacon slices

2 boneless pork chops, each cut into 4 strips

2 tablespoons extra-virgin olive oil

1. Wrap 1 bacon slice around a pork strip and secure with a toothpick. Repeat with the remaining bacon and pork strips.

2. In a skillet, heat the olive oil over medium-high heat.

3. Add the bacon-wrapped nuggets and cook on each side for 5 minutes, until the bacon is crispy. Using tongs, flip the strips on their sides and sear the bacon until crispy all the way around.

4. Place the finished nuggets on a paper towel–lined plate to cool before serving.

Variation: I like to dip these in ranch or blue cheese dressing, but sugar-free barbecue sauce and Dairy-Free Avocado Crema (page 257) are also great options.

MACRONUTRIENTS	76.5% FAT	23% PROTEIN	.5% CARBS

CALORIES: 353; TOTAL FAT: 30G; PROTEIN: 20G; TOTAL CARBS: 1G; FIBER: 0G; NET CARBS: 1G

BACON-CAULIFLOWER MAC AND CHEESE

PREP TIME: 10 MINUTES **COOK TIME:** 20 MINUTES

There's no need to miss mac and cheese on keto—just make this decadent version instead. Your family will love this whether they are keto or not. As a great meal or hearty side dish, this is what I always find myself craving on chilly nights. *Serves 2*

○ COMFORT FOOD
● NUT-FREE
○ SUPER QUICK

4 bacon slices

½ cauliflower head, cut into florets

Salt

Freshly ground black pepper

¼ cup heavy whipping cream

2 tablespoons crumbled goat cheese

1 teaspoon Dijon mustard

¾ cup shredded Cheddar cheese

Nonstick cooking spray

¼ cup shredded Gruyère cheese

1. Preheat the oven to 375°F.

2. In a large skillet, cook the bacon over medium-high heat for about 8 minutes, flipping once, until crispy. Transfer the bacon to a paper towel–lined plate to drain and cool, then crumble it.

3. While the bacon is cooking, fill a medium saucepan half full with water and bring to a boil over high heat. Add the cauliflower and cook for 4 minutes. Drain the cauliflower and place it on a paper towel–lined plate. Using paper towels or a clean, dry kitchen towel, pat the florets to remove as much water as possible. Season with salt and pepper.

4. Return the saucepan to the burner and add the heavy cream, goat cheese, and Dijon over medium heat, whisking until smooth. Add the Cheddar cheese and whisk again until the cheese melts.

5. Spray a small baking dish with cooking spray. Add the cauliflower and pour the cheese sauce on top. Add a layer of crumbled bacon and top with the Gruyère cheese.

6. Bake for 15 minutes, or until golden and bubbling.

Variation: Cheddar, cream cheese, and Parmesan is also a great combination. Replace the goat cheese with cream cheese, the Gruyère with extra Cheddar, and sprinkle Parmesan on top.

MACRONUTRIENTS	75% FAT	19% PROTEIN	6% CARBS

CALORIES: 636; TOTAL FAT: 54G; PROTEIN: 30G; TOTAL CARBS: 10G; FIBER: 4G; NET CARBS: 6G

CRISPY OVEN-BAKED PORK BELLY

PREP TIME: 5 MINUTES **COOK TIME:** 40 MINUTES

Pork belly is a perfect keto food and is really easy to make. You want to add lots of salt to get the skin nice and crispy. Cut it up and add it on top of any number of dishes, or just enjoy it all by itself. *Serves 2*

● ALLERGEN-FREE
○ COMFORT FOOD
● DAIRY-FREE
● NUT-FREE
● PALEO OR PALEO-FRIENDLY

½ pound pork belly

1 tablespoon extra-virgin olive oil

½ tablespoon salt

Freshly ground black pepper

1. Preheat the oven to 450°F.

2. Pat the pork belly dry and score the skin with a sharp knife. I score every ½ inch.

3. Place the pork belly on a wire rack in a roasting pan.

4. Rub the skin on all sides with the olive oil and then rub the salt onto both sides. Season with pepper.

5. Roast for 35 minutes on the middle rack of the oven.

6. Adjust the oven to the broil setting and move an oven shelf as close to the broiler as possible.

7. Broil for 1 minute and check on the pork belly. You want the skin to be bubbling, puffy, and golden brown. Once that has happened, remove the pan from the broiler and let the pork belly rest for 10 minutes. Slice and serve.

Variation: To get the skin of the pork belly extra dry before roasting, you can season it with salt and pepper and leave it uncovered in the refrigerator overnight.

MACRONUTRIENTS	93% FAT	7% PROTEIN	0% CARBS

CALORIES: 647; TOTAL FAT: 67G; PROTEIN: 11G; TOTAL CARBS: 0G; FIBER: 0G; NET CARBS: 0G

BACON-WRAPPED PORK LOIN

PREP TIME: 10 MINUTES **COOK TIME:** 1 HOUR

Pork loin is so easy to make, and this one is no exception. Feel free to add veggies to the pan if you want, and roast them at the same time as the pork loin. This dish makes more than two servings because I can never seem to find a pork loin smaller than 2 pounds, but if you can find one and want a smaller portion, feel free to adjust! *Serves 6*

- ● ALLERGEN-FREE
- ○ COMFORT FOOD
- ◐ DAIRY-FREE
- ● NUT-FREE
- ● PALEO OR PALEO-FRIENDLY

1 (2-pound) pork loin

Salt

Freshly ground black pepper

8 bacon slices (thin slices work best)

1. Preheat the oven to 375°F.

2. Pat the pork loin dry and season with salt and pepper. Place the loin in a baking dish and, using a sharp knife, score the top of the meat.

3. Wrap the bacon slices horizontally across the top of the pork loin.

4. Bake for 1 hour, or until the bacon is crispy and the meat is cooked through.

5. Allow the pork loin to rest for 15 minutes before slicing.

Variation: Broccoli, cauliflower, Brussels sprouts, and mushrooms are all great veggie options if you wish to add them to the baking dish.

MACRONUTRIENTS	68% FAT	32% PROTEIN	0% CARBS

CALORIES: 447; TOTAL FAT: 34G; PROTEIN: 33G; TOTAL CARBS: 0G; FIBER: 0G; NET CARBS: 0G

PORK BUTTER BURGER

PREP TIME: 10 MINUTES **COOK TIME:** 15 MINUTES

A burger stuffed with butter?! How could that not be delicious? If you haven't used ground pork for a burger before, you are in for a treat! Make your herb butter ahead of time so it starts out nice and hard. Your burgers will be juicy and full of flavor. *Serves 2*

○ COMFORT FOOD
● NUT-FREE
○ SUPER QUICK

½ pound ground pork

Salt

Freshly ground black pepper

4 tablespoons Herby Butter (page 30), divided

2 slices Gruyère cheese

1. Heat a large skillet over medium-high heat.

2. In a medium bowl, season the ground pork with salt and pepper and create 2 patties.

3. Stuff 1 tablespoon of herby butter into the middle of each patty, then cover the butter with the meat. Pack the patties firmly, as pork burgers are more delicate than beef while cooking.

4. Add the burgers to the hot skillet and then add 1 additional tablespoon of herby butter on top of each patty. Cook the burgers for 7 to 8 minutes on each side, flipping once.

5. Add a slice of cheese to the top of each patty at the very end and melt.

Variation: This recipe also works great with ground beef.

MACRONUTRIENTS	79% FAT	21% PROTEIN	0% CARBS

CALORIES: 504; TOTAL FAT: 44G; PROTEIN: 27G; TOTAL CARBS: 0G; FIBER: 0G; NET CARBS: 0G

PORK BURGER LETTUCE CUPS

PREP TIME: 10 MINUTES **COOK TIME:** 15 MINUTES

I love a slider, and these are nestled in butter lettuce cups, which makes them easy to eat and super fresh when mixed with thinly sliced red onions and radishes. The freshness mixed with the savory ground pork is the perfect combination. *Serves 2*

● ALLERGEN-FREE
○ COMFORT FOOD
◐ DAIRY-FREE
● NUT-FREE
● PALEO OR PALEO-FRIENDLY
○ SUPER QUICK

1 tablespoon extra-virgin olive oil

½ pound ground pork

Salt

Freshly ground black pepper

2 teaspoons Sriracha, divided

1 tablespoon avocado oil mayonnaise

4 butter lettuce leaves

¼ cup thinly sliced red onion

2 radishes, thinly sliced

2 lime wedges

1. In a large skillet, heat the olive oil over medium-high heat.

2. In a medium bowl, season the ground pork with salt and pepper and 1 teaspoon of Sriracha. Create four slider-size patties. Pack them firmly, as pork burgers are more delicate than beef while cooking.

3. Add the burgers to the skillet, and cook for 7 to 8 minutes on each side.

4. In a small bowl, combine the mayonnaise with the remaining 1 teaspoon of Sriracha and mix well.

5. Place 2 lettuce leaves on each plate. Add the onions, radishes, and a slider in each lettuce cup. Place a dollop of Sriracha mayonnaise on top and squeeze lime wedges over each one.

Variation: Thinly sliced cucumbers and carrots also make great additions.

MACRONUTRIENTS	75% FAT	21% PROTEIN	4% CARBS

CALORIES: 395; TOTAL FAT: 33G; PROTEIN: 20G; TOTAL CARBS: 5G; FIBER: 1G; NET CARBS: 4G

PARMESAN-CRUSTED PORK CHOPS

PREP TIME: 10 MINUTES **COOK TIME:** 10 MINUTES

I love using pork rinds as a faux bread crumb, and this dish is
a fun variation to make a perfectly crisp and flavorful pork chop.
I use boneless pork chops because they are affordable and cook
quickly on a busy night. *Serves 2*

○ COMFORT FOOD
● NUT-FREE
○ SUPER QUICK

1 large egg

¼ cup grated Parmesan cheese

¼ cup Pork Rind "Bread" Crumbs
(page 249)

½ teaspoon Italian Seasoning
(page 246)

2 boneless pork chops

Salt

Freshly ground black pepper

1 tablespoon extra-virgin olive oil

1. In a small bowl, beat the egg. On a plate, mix the
   Parmesan cheese, pork rinds, and Italian seasoning.

2. Pat the pork chops dry and season with salt and
   pepper. Then dip each chop in the egg and press
   into the Parmesan-pork rind mixture.

3. In a large skillet, heat the olive oil over medium heat.
   Add the pork chops and cook for 4 to 5 minutes per
   side, flipping once.

4. Let the pork chops rest for 10 minutes before serving.

Variation: For some acidity, ¼ teaspoon of lemon or lime zest
is a nice addition to the Parmesan–pork rind mixture.

MACRONUTRIENTS	66% FAT	34% PROTEIN	0% CARBS

CALORIES: 395; TOTAL FAT: 29G; PROTEIN: 31G; TOTAL CARBS: 1G; FIBER: 0; NET CARBS: 1G

HERB AND DIJON PORK CHOPS

PREP TIME: 10 MINUTES **COOK TIME:** 17 MINUTES

Dijon mustard and Parmesan cheese add a delicious bite to these pork chops. Mixed with the mayonnaise, the creamy combination keeps the pork chops juicy and full of flavor. *Serves 2*

○ COMFORT FOOD
● NUT-FREE
○ SUPER QUICK

1 tablespoon Dijon mustard

1 tablespoon avocado oil mayonnaise

½ teaspoon Italian Seasoning (page 246)

Salt

Freshly ground black pepper

2 boneless pork chops

¼ cup grated Parmesan cheese

1 teaspoon minced fresh parsley

1. Preheat the oven to 400°F.

2. In a bowl, mix the Dijon, mayonnaise, and Italian seasoning. Season with salt and pepper.

3. Pat the pork chops dry and season with salt and pepper. Place in a baking dish.

4. Spread the Dijon-mayonnaise mixture on the pork chops and sprinkle the Parmesan cheese on top.

5. Bake for 15 minutes.

6. Adjust the oven to broil and cook for 1 to 2 minutes, until golden.

7. Let the pork chops rest for 10 minutes, sprinkle the parsley on top, and serve.

Variation: The Dijon-mayonnaise mixture can also act as a marinade for the pork chops. Marinate for a few hours or even a full day. Then just sprinkle the Parmesan on before baking.

| MACRONUTRIENTS | 61% FAT | 36% PROTEIN | 3% CARBS |

CALORIES: 323; TOTAL FAT: 22G; PROTEIN: 27G; TOTAL CARBS: 3G; FIBER: 0G; NET CARBS: 3G

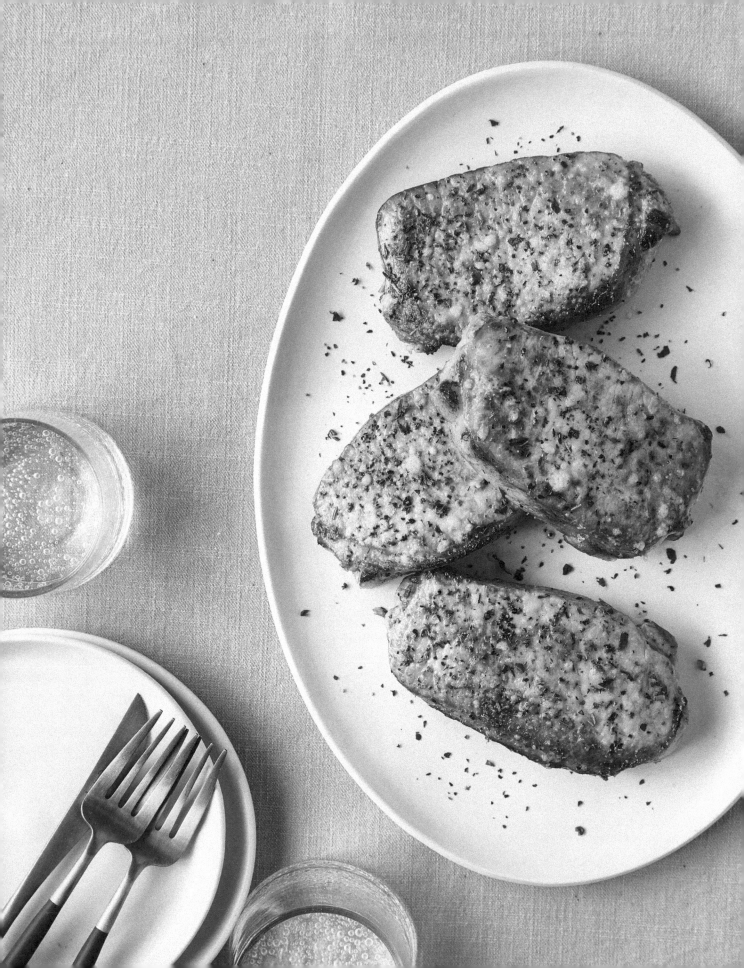

CREAMY PORK CHOPS

PREP TIME: 5 MINUTES **COOK TIME:** 20 MINUTES

Ranch seasoning is one of my go-tos because it adds a nice tang to pretty much any kind of meat or fish. This recipe adds ranch seasoning and one of my other favorite things, cream cheese, to create a delicious fatty sauce over pork chops. *Serves 2*

○ COMFORT FOOD
● NUT-FREE
○ SUPER QUICK

2 boneless pork chops

Salt

Freshly ground black pepper

2 tablespoons butter or ghee

1 tablespoon chicken broth or chicken bone broth

2 ounces cream cheese or Dairy-Free Cream Cheese (page 258)

1 tablespoon Ranch Seasoning (page 248)

1. Pat the pork chops dry and season with salt and pepper.

2. In a large skillet, melt the butter over medium-high heat.

3. Add the pork chops and cook for 4 to 5 minutes per side, flipping once. Transfer to a plate.

4. Reduce the heat to medium and add the chicken broth to deglaze the skillet, scraping up all the brown bits. Add the cream cheese and ranch seasoning. Stir or whisk until the mixture is completely combined.

5. Reduce the heat to low, add the pork chops back into the sauce, and simmer for 10 minutes.

6. Let the pork chops rest for 10 minutes before serving.

Make It Paleo: Use Dairy-Free Cream Cheese (page 258) in place of the cream cheese.

MACRONUTRIENTS	75% FAT	24% PROTEIN	1% CARBS

CALORIES: 432; TOTAL FAT: 37G; PROTEIN: 24G; TOTAL CARBS: 1G; FIBER: 0G; NET CARBS: 1G

BUTTERY SLOW COOKER PORK LOIN

PREP TIME: 5 MINUTES **COOK TIME:** 8 HOURS

So easy, so yummy. I never tire of an easy slow cooker meal. If you can't find a 1-pound pork loin, just buy a larger one and you'll have delicious leftovers! You're going to love how your house smells when this is cooking! *Serves 2*

○ COMFORT FOOD
● NUT-FREE

1 (1-pound) pork loin

Salt

Freshly ground black pepper

1 garlic clove, minced

2 teaspoons Italian Seasoning (page 246)

½ teaspoon red pepper flakes

2 tablespoons butter or ghee

1. Preheat the slow cooker on low.

2. Pat the pork loin dry with paper towels and season with salt and pepper.

3. In the slow cooker, add the pork loin and top it with the garlic, Italian seasoning, red pepper flakes, and butter.

4. Cover the slow cooker and cook for 8 hours. Slice and serve.

Variation: If you are in a rush, you can cook this for 4 hours on high instead.

MACRONUTRIENTS	46% FAT	54% PROTEIN	0% CARBS

CALORIES: 372; TOTAL FAT: 19G; PROTEIN: 47G; TOTAL CARBS: 1G; FIBER: 0G; NET CARBS: 1G

DOUBLE PORK CHOPS

PREP TIME: 10 MINUTES **COOK TIME:** 10 MINUTES

These pork chops are so crispy on the outside and super moist on the inside, you will love them! You've probably noticed I love using pork rind "bread" crumbs. I have tricked many non-keto people into thinking they are actual bread crumbs, but in my opinion they are even better. Pair them with a fresh side like the Avocado Cotija Salad (page 109) for a great meal. *Serves 2*

○ COMFORT FOOD
◑ DAIRY-FREE
● NUT-FREE
● PALEO OR PALEO-FRIENDLY
○ SUPER QUICK

1 large egg

½ cup coconut flour

1 teaspoon cayenne pepper

Salt

Freshly ground black pepper

½ cup Pork Rind "Bread" Crumbs (page 249)

2 tablespoons extra-virgin olive oil or ghee

2 boneless pork chops

1. In a small bowl, lightly beat the egg. On a large plate, mix the coconut flour and cayenne pepper. Season with salt and pepper. On another large plate, add the pork rind "bread" crumbs.

2. In a large skillet, heat the olive oil over medium-high heat.

3. Dredge each pork chop on both sides in the coconut flour mixture. Dip the pork chops into the egg, coating both sides. Dredge the pork chops in the crushed pork rinds, pressing the pork rinds into the pork chop so they stick. Place the pork chops in the hot skillet.

4. Cook for 4 to 5 minutes on each side, until the pork chops are golden, crispy, and cooked through.

Variation: Additional seasoning can be added to the pork rind "bread" crumbs if you want to make them spicy. I like to add a teaspoon of Ranch Seasoning (page 248).

MACRONUTRIENTS	56% FAT	28% PROTEIN	16% CARBS

CALORIES: 483; TOTAL FAT: 30G; PROTEIN: 31G; TOTAL CARBS: 19G; FIBER: 12G; NET CARBS: 7G

SRIRACHA PORK STIR-FRY

PREP TIME: 5 MINUTES **COOK TIME:** 20 MINUTES

This quick stir-fry came about one night when I had very limited food in my refrigerator. What I discovered that night is that you can add Sriracha to pretty much anything and it will make it better! Ground pork is a nice alternative to ground beef for burgers and for stir-fries like this. *Serves 2*

● ALLERGEN-FREE
○ COMFORT FOOD
◐ DAIRY-FREE
● NUT-FREE
● PALEO OR PALEO-FRIENDLY
○ SUPER QUICK

2 tablespoons sesame oil, divided

½ pound ground pork

1 garlic clove, minced

½ onion, diced

½ bell pepper, cut into strips

¼ pound asparagus, cut into 1- to 2-inch pieces

2 teaspoons Sriracha

2 tablespoons soy sauce or coconut aminos

¼ cup chopped cilantro

1. In a large skillet, heat 1 tablespoon of sesame oil over medium-high heat. Add the pork and cook for 8 to 10 minutes, breaking it into smaller pieces as it cooks, until it is browned completely. Remove from the pan and set aside.

2. In the skillet, add the remaining 1 tablespoon of sesame oil as well as the garlic and onion, and sauté for about 3 minutes, until softened. Add the bell pepper and asparagus and cook for 3 to 4 minutes, stirring occasionally.

3. Add the Sriracha, soy sauce, and pork to the skillet and mix well.

4. Divide between two bowls and top with the cilantro.

Variation: Cauliflower rice or shirataki rice is a great addition to this dish and makes it very filling.

MACRONUTRIENTS	72% FAT	20% PROTEIN	8% CARBS

CALORIES: 469; TOTAL FAT: 38G; PROTEIN: 24G; TOTAL CARBS: 11G; FIBER: 4G; NET CARBS: 7G

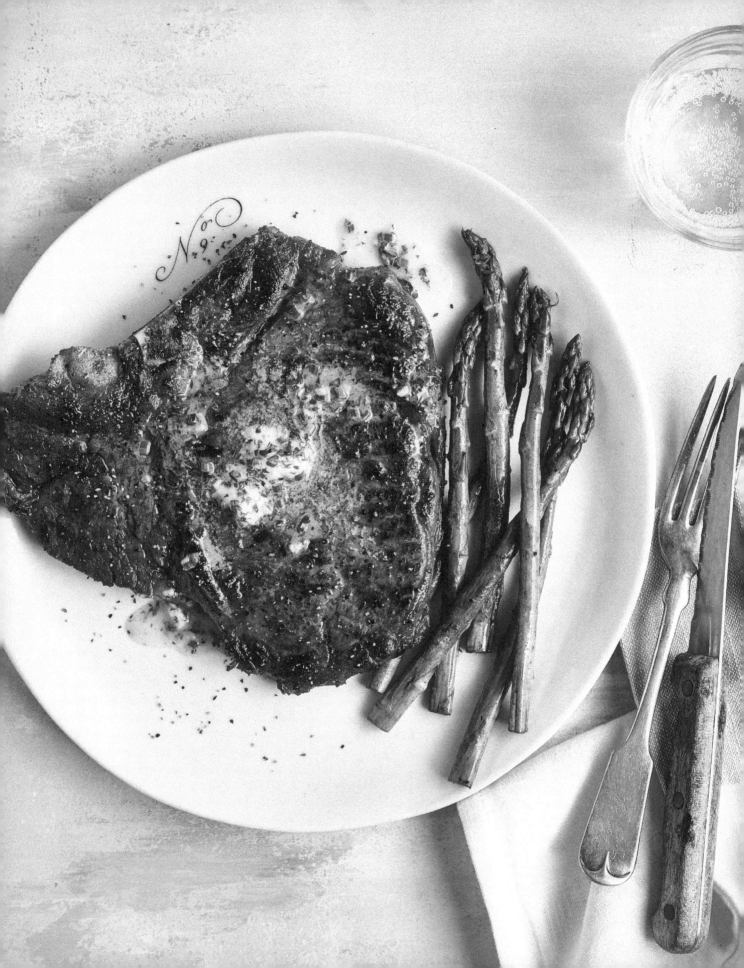

BEEF

CHAPTER ELEVEN

Opposite: Pan-Seared T-Bone Steak with Herby Butter

PAN-SEARED T-BONE STEAK
WITH HERBY BUTTER

PREP TIME: 15 MINUTES, PLUS 30 MINUTES TO SET STEAKS OUT   **COOK TIME:** 18 TO 20 MINUTES

Some nights you just want a big juicy steak! You can make this on the grill if you prefer, but I don't have a grill, so I make mine in a skillet and it comes out great. *Serves 2*

○ COMFORT FOOD
● NUT-FREE

1 (12-ounce) T-bone steak

2 tablespoons extra-virgin olive oil or avocado oil

Salt and pepper

4 tablespoons Herby Butter (page 30)

1. Set your steak on the counter for 30 minutes to bring it to room temperature.

2. Heat an oven-proof skillet over high heat for 5 minutes— you want it to be searing hot.

3. Preheat the oven to 400°F.

4. While the skillet heats, rub the steak with olive oil. Season both sides with salt and pepper.

5. Add the oiled and seasoned steak to the skillet and sear for 3 minutes. Turn the steak over with tongs and sear the other side for 2 minutes.

6. Place the herby butter under the steak and put the skillet in the oven. If your skillet is not oven safe, put the butter on a baking sheet and place the steak on top.

7. I cook my steak for 8 minutes, or until it reaches about 140°F because I like my steak between medium-rare and medium.

8. Pull the cooked steak out of the oven, place it on a plate, and loosely tent with aluminum foil. Allow the steak to rest for 5 to 10 minutes.

9. Top with Herby Butter just before serving.

Variation: Measuring with a meat thermometer, cook your steak until the internal temperature reaches your desired doneness: 125°F is rare, 135°F is medium-rare, 145°F is medium, 155°F is medium-well, and 165°F is well done.

MACRONUTRIENTS	79% FAT	21% PROTEIN	0% CARBS

CALORIES: 854; TOTAL FAT: 75G; PROTEIN: 45G; TOTAL CARBS: 0.5G; FIBER: 0G; NET CARBS: 0.5G

SLOW COOKER STEAK AND MUSHROOM BITES

PREP TIME: 5 MINUTES **COOK TIME:** 6 HOURS

Easy, full of flavor, and absolutely delicious, this is one of my favorite slow cooker dishes. I like to serve it over cauliflower rice. It requires just 5 minutes of prep time. Then let let it cook all day, and you have an incredible meal. *Serves 2*

○ COMFORT FOOD

◐ DAIRY-FREE

● NUT-FREE

● PALEO OR PALEO-FRIENDLY

6 tablespoons butter or ghee

1 tablespoon Ranch Seasoning (page 248)

1 (¾-pound) skirt steak, cut into bite-size pieces

8 ounces mushrooms, cremini or button

1 tablespoon chopped fresh parsley

1. Preheat the slow cooker on low.

2. In the slow cooker, add the butter and ranch seasoning. Once the butter is melted, mix well.

3. Add the steak and mushrooms to the slow cooker.

4. Cover and cook for 6 hours.

5. Divide between two plates and top with the parsley.

MACRONUTRIENTS	78% FAT	20% PROTEIN	2% CARBS

CALORIES: 594; TOTAL FAT: 52G; PROTEIN: 29G; TOTAL CARBS: 5G; FIBER: 1G; NET CARBS: 4G

SLOW COOKER CHILI

PREP TIME: 15 MINUTES **COOK TIME:** 8 HOURS

This keto version of chili has all the flavor of chili without the beans. The vegetables provide a great depth to the texture. I love using the tomatoes that already have the green chiles chopped in them, as well as the extra seasoning the pickled jalapeño peppers add. *Serves 4*

● DAIRY-FREE
● NUT-FREE
● PALEO OR PALEO-FRIENDLY

1 pound ground beef

1 garlic clove, minced

Salt

Freshly ground black pepper

½ onion, diced

2 celery stalks, chopped

1 (10-ounce) can diced tomatoes and green chiles

2 tablespoons tomato paste

2 tablespoons Taco Seasoning (page 245)

2 tablespoons soy sauce or coconut aminos

1 sliced jalapeño pepper or 2 tablespoons pickled jalapeño peppers

¼ cup shredded Mexican blend cheese (optional)

2 tablespoons sour cream (optional)

4 cooked bacon slices, crumbled (optional)

¼ cup sliced scallions, green parts only (optional)

1. Preheat the slow cooker on low.

2. In a large skillet, cook the ground beef and garlic over medium-high heat. Season with salt and pepper and cook for 6 to 7 minutes, breaking it apart as it cooks, until browned. Drain any excess fat and transfer the ground beef to the slow cooker.

3. In the slow cooker, add the onion, celery, tomatoes and their juices, tomato paste, taco seasoning, soy sauce, and jalapeño pepper. Mix well.

4. Cover and cook for 8 hours.

5. Divide the chili into bowls and top with your preferred optional toppings: shredded cheese, sour cream, crumbled bacon, and/or scallions.

Make Ahead: Chili is excellent reheated—maybe even better the second time because all the flavors soak together longer. You can add beef broth or bone broth to thin it out a bit for reheating.

MACRONUTRIENTS (WITH TOPPINGS)	61% FAT	30% PROTEIN	9% CARBS

CALORIES: 399; TOTAL FAT: 27G; PROTEIN: 30G; TOTAL CARBS: 9G; FIBER: 1G; NET CARBS: 8G

FAJITA-SPICED SKIRT STEAK
WITH MEXICAN CAULIFLOWER RICE

PREP TIME: 15 MINUTES, PLUS 30 MINUTES OR MORE TO MARINATE **COOK TIME:** 15 MINUTES

Skirt steak is one of my favorite cuts of meat, as it takes on so much flavor. I don't have a grill, so I cook it in a skillet over high heat to get a nice sear. Cutting thin slices against the grain is my favorite way to serve it over salads, in tacos, or in this case, over cauliflower rice. *Serves 2*

- ● ALLERGEN-FREE
- ○ COMFORT FOOD
- ◐ DAIRY-FREE
- ● NUT-FREE
- ● PALEO OR PALEO-FRIENDLY

FOR THE SKIRT STEAK

1 garlic clove, peeled

½ onion, roughly chopped

1 tablespoon freshly squeezed lime juice

1 tablespoon chopped cilantro

½ bell pepper

½ jalapeño pepper, seeded, stemmed, and ribs removed

3 tablespoons extra-virgin olive oil

Salt

Freshly ground black pepper

½ pound skirt steak

TO MAKE THE SKIRT STEAK

1. In a food processor, combine the garlic, onion, lime juice, cilantro, bell pepper, jalapeño pepper, and olive oil, and process until smooth. Season with salt and pepper. Transfer to a resealable bag or bowl, place the skirt steak in the marinade, and refrigerate for at least 30 minutes or up to a day in advance.

2. In a skillet over high heat, add the skirt steak and sear on each side for 3 minutes.

3. Let the meat rest for 10 minutes before slicing.

4. Slice against the grain; otherwise, the meat will be tough. I also like to cut it at a sharp angle.

continued

MACRONUTRIENTS	58% FAT	29% PROTEIN	13% CARBS

CALORIES: 355; TOTAL FAT: 23G; PROTEIN: 26G; TOTAL CARBS: 11G; FIBER: 4G; NET CARBS: 7G

FAJITA-SPICED SKIRT STEAK WITH MEXICAN CAULIFLOWER RICE, CONTINUED

FOR THE CAULIFLOWER RICE

1 tablespoon extra-virgin olive oil

½ jalapeño pepper, seeded and sliced

1 garlic clove, minced

½ cup diced onion

¼ cup diced bell pepper

2 cups cauliflower, riced

1 teaspoon Chili-Lime Seasoning (page 244)

1 tablespoon chopped cilantro

2 lime wedges

TO MAKE THE CAULIFLOWER RICE

1. While the meat rests, wipe the skillet clean and heat the olive oil over medium heat. Add the jalapeño pepper, garlic, and onion. Cook until softened, stirring occasionally.

2. Add the bell pepper, cauliflower rice, and chili-lime seasoning and mix well.

3. Cook for 5 minutes, stirring regularly, until the cauliflower is softened.

4. Remove the skillet from the heat, mix in the cilantro, and squeeze the lime over the cauliflower.

Variation: If you are looking for a vegetarian meal or great side dish, you can skip the steak and just make the Mexican cauliflower rice!

SHEET PAN FAJITAS

PREP TIME: 15 MINUTES, PLUS 30 MINUTES OR MORE TO MARINATE **COOK TIME:** 20 MINUTES

This recipe uses the same marinade as the last dish, the Fajita-Spiced Skirt Steak with Mexican Cauliflower Rice (page 185), but the steak is prepared in the oven and the marinade pulls double duty, providing great flavor to the steak and the veggies. *Serves 2*

- ● ALLERGEN-FREE
- ○ COMFORT FOOD
- ◐ DAIRY-FREE
- ● NUT-FREE
- ● PALEO OR PALEO-FRIENDLY

FOR THE SKIRT STEAK

1 garlic clove, peeled

½ onion, roughly chopped

1 tablespoon freshly squeezed lime juice

1 tablespoon chopped cilantro

½ bell pepper

½ jalapeño pepper, seeded, stemmed, and ribs removed

3 tablespoons extra-virgin olive oil

Salt

Freshly ground black pepper

½ pound skirt steak

FOR THE FAJITAS

1½ bell peppers, cut into strips

½ onion, cut into strips

2 lime wedges

TO MAKE THE SKIRT STEAK

In a food processor, combine the garlic, onion, lime juice, cilantro, bell pepper, jalapeño pepper, and olive oil, and process until smooth. Season with salt and pepper. Transfer to a resealable bag or bowl, place the skirt steak in the marinade, and refrigerate for at least 30 minutes or up to a day in advance.

TO MAKE THE FAJITAS

1. Preheat the oven to 425°F.
2. On a large baking sheet, arrange the bell peppers and onion in a single layer, leaving a space in the middle for the steak. Nestle the steak in the middle of the baking sheet and then pour the marinade over the steak and veggies.
3. Bake for 20 minutes.
4. Heat a dry skillet over high heat. Add the skirt steak and sear on each side for 3 minutes.
5. Let the meat rest for 10 minutes.
6. Slice against the grain; otherwise, the meat will be tough. I also like to cut it at a sharp angle.

Variation: You can serve the meat and veggies as your full meal or add it to low-carb tortillas and top with avocado and sour cream.

MACRONUTRIENTS	63% FAT	24% PROTEIN	13% CARBS

CALORIES: 426; TOTAL FAT: 30G; PROTEIN: 26G; TOTAL CARBS: 13G; FIBER: 3G; NET CARBS: 10G

ASIAN BEEF "NOODLE" BOWLS

PREP TIME: 10 MINUTES **COOK TIME:** 10 MINUTES

The Asian flavors in this dish make me think of takeout in all the right ways. Salty, savory, and with a nice kick, this quick one-skillet dish is packed with flavors. You can choose what variety of keto-friendly "noodles" you want to add. In this recipe, I use fettuccine-style shirataki noodles. *Serves 2*

○ COMFORT FOOD

◐ DAIRY-FREE

● NUT-FREE

● PALEO OR PALEO-FRIENDLY

○ SUPER QUICK

2 tablespoons sesame oil, divided

1 celery stalk, diced

1 tablespoon peeled, grated fresh ginger

1 garlic clove, minced

½ pound ground beef

Salt

Freshly ground black pepper

1 tablespoon Sriracha

1 teaspoon fish sauce

1 tablespoon freshly squeezed lime juice

1 tablespoon soy sauce or coconut aminos

1 batch Shirataki Noodles (page 40)

1 Persian cucumber, sliced thin (or ½ cucumber)

2 tablespoons sliced scallions, green parts only

1 tablespoon sesame seeds

1. In a large skillet, heat 1 tablespoon of sesame oil over medium-high heat. Add the celery, ginger, and garlic and cook for 1 minute, stirring frequently.

2. Add the beef and season with salt and pepper. Cook for 6 to 7 minutes, until browned.

3. Meanwhile, in a small bowl, combine the remaining 1 tablespoon of sesame oil, and the Sriracha, fish sauce, lime juice, and soy sauce.

4. Pour the sauce over the meat, reduce the heat to medium, and let the meat simmer in the sauce for 1 minute.

5. Push the meat to one side of the skillet, add the shirataki noodles, and cook for 1 minute so they take on the flavor of the sauce. Toss all the ingredients together in the pan.

6. Divide between two bowls and top with the sliced cucumbers, scallions, and sesame seeds.

Variation: Typically, Asian marinades include sugar. This one has been keto-fied, so it does not, but you can add a pinch of erythritol if you wish.

MACRONUTRIENTS	69% FAT	24% PROTEIN	7% CARBS

CALORIES: 404; TOTAL FAT: 31G; PROTEIN: 25G; TOTAL CARBS: 9G; FIBER: 2G; NET CARBS: 7G

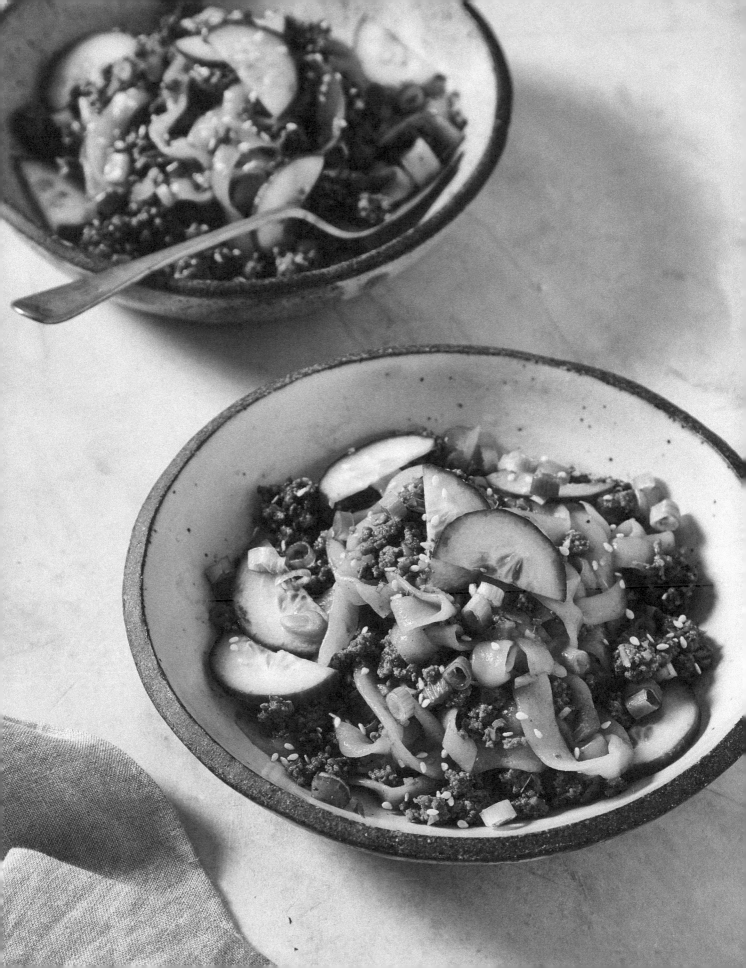

OVEN-BAKED GARLIC AND HERB STEAK

PREP TIME: 15 MINUTES **COOK TIME:** 20 MINUTES

There is something that feels fancy about steak with herb butter
on top, like you're at a steakhouse where they charge you extra to
get the special butter. This one is super simple. It's so good I could
eat it with a spoon. *Serves 2*

○ COMFORT FOOD

● NUT-FREE

8 radishes, halved

1 bell pepper, diced

¼ cup diced onion

1 tablespoon extra-virgin olive oil

Salt

Freshly ground black pepper

1 (12-ounce) sirloin steak, cut into
2-inch cubes

1 batch Herby Butter (page 30)

1. Preheat the oven to 425°F.

2. In a small bowl, toss the radishes, bell pepper, onion,
   and olive oil. Season with salt and pepper and mix well.

3. In another small bowl, season the steak with salt
   and pepper.

4. Cut two sheets of aluminum foil into 12-by-12-inch
   squares. Place half the vegetables in the center of each
   piece of foil and top with the steak pieces and herb
   butter. Seal the foil packets by crimping the edges
   together, and place them on a baking sheet.

5. Cook for 18 minutes. Adjust the oven to broil, carefully
   open the foil packets, and cook for 3 more minutes. Serve.

Variation: If you like more of a sear on your steak, you can sear
the steak pieces before baking and skip the broiling step.

MACRONUTRIENTS	71% FAT	25% PROTEIN	4% CARBS

CALORIES: 609; TOTAL FAT: 48G; PROTEIN: 36G; TOTAL CARBS: 6G; FIBER: 2G; NET CARBS: 4G

VIETNAMESE STEAK AND CAULIFLOWER RICE BOWL

PREP TIME: 15 MINUTES **COOK TIME:** 10 MINUTES

I used to be intimidated by steak and would order it only at restaurants instead of making it at home. Then I started making dishes like this one and realized how quick and simple it really is to prepare. *Serves 2*

- ● ALLERGEN-FREE
- ○ COMFORT FOOD
- ◐ DAIRY-FREE
- ● NUT-FREE
- ● PALEO OR PALEO-FRIENDLY

1 jalapeño pepper, sliced

2 tablespoons extra-virgin olive oil, divided

2 tablespoons soy sauce or coconut aminos

½ lime, juiced, divided

1 garlic clove, minced

Salt

Freshly ground black pepper

1 (12-ounce) sirloin steak

1 (7-ounce) package shirataki rice or 1 batch Cauliflower Rice (page 36)

1 cucumber, thinly sliced

4 radishes, thinly sliced

1 tablespoon fresh mint, cut into ribbons

1. In a medium bowl, combine the jalapeño pepper, 1 tablespoon of olive oil, the soy sauce, half the lime juice, and the garlic. Season with salt and pepper.

2. Slice the steak into two thinner steaks to allow it to cook faster and take in more flavor. Place the cut steaks into the bowl with the marinade.

3. While the steaks are marinating, cook the shirataki rice according to the package instructions.

4. In a small bowl, toss the cucumber and radishes with the remaining lime juice and season with salt and pepper.

5. In a skillet, heat the remaining 1 tablespoon of olive oil over high heat. Add the steak and sear on each side for 2 to 2½ minutes.

6. Allow the cooked steak to rest for a few minutes. Toss the shirataki rice with the mint and the cucumber-radish mixture and divide between two bowls.

7. Slice the steak against the grain and place on top of the shirataki rice and vegetables in the bowls.

Variation: If you want extra spice, add sliced jalapeño peppers to the cucumber and radish. You can also add erythritol (to taste) if you want to counteract the spicy and sour with a bit of sweet.

MACRONUTRIENTS	66% FAT	29% PROTEIN	5% CARBS

CALORIES: 466; TOTAL FAT: 34G; PROTEIN: 34G; TOTAL CARBS: 6G; FIBER: 1G; NET CARBS: 5G

SHEET PAN STEAK AND EGGS

PREP TIME: 10 MINUTES **COOK TIME:** 10 MINUTES

In my opinion, steak and eggs is a great meal any time of day! Here, gooey eggs mix with steak and spinach for a quick, easy, and delicious meal. This is a great dish to double or triple for a large group. *Serves 2*

○ COMFORT FOOD
◐ DAIRY-FREE
● NUT-FREE
● PALEO OR PALEO-FRIENDLY
○ SUPER QUICK

1 (8-ounce) sirloin steak

Salt

Freshly ground black pepper

2 tablespoons butter or ghee

8 ounces spinach

2 large eggs

1. Preheat the oven on broil.

2. Season the steak with salt and pepper.

3. Place the steak in the middle of a large baking sheet. Broil for 4 minutes.

4. Remove the baking sheet from the oven, flip the steak, and top it with the butter.

5. Arrange the spinach in two mounds next to the steak on the baking sheet and create a well in the center of each for the eggs.

6. Crack 1 egg into each well and season it with salt and pepper.

7. Broil for 4 to 5 more minutes, until the eggs are set.

Variation: Sprinkle Parmesan cheese on top of the spinach and eggs for the last minute of broiling.

MACRONUTRIENTS	64% FAT	32% PROTEIN	4% CARBS

CALORIES: 409; TOTAL FAT: 29G; PROTEIN: 33G; TOTAL CARBS: 4G; FIBER: 2G; NET CARBS: 2G

MEDITERRANEAN BURGER

PREP TIME: 10 MINUTES **COOK TIME:** 15 MINUTES

I love egg bakes that feature feta and spinach, so I figured I would do a take on that with this burger. I'm using ground beef and pork combined for extra flavor. I like to eat each bite of burger with a little grape tomato, spinach, and runny egg. *Serves 2*

○ COMFORT FOOD
● NUT-FREE
○ SUPER QUICK

¼ pound ground pork

¼ pound ground beef

2 tablespoons sliced scallions, green parts only

Salt

Freshly ground black pepper

¼ cup crumbled feta cheese

2 tablespoons extra-virgin olive oil, divided

2 large eggs

8 ounces spinach

½ cup grape tomatoes, halved

1. In a medium bowl, combine the pork, beef, and scallions. Season with salt and pepper and mix well.

2. Create two large patties with indentations in the middle. Fill the indentations with the feta and then seal with meat.

3. In a large skillet, heat 1 tablespoon of olive oil over medium heat. Add the burger patties and cook on each side for 4 to 5 minutes, until cooked through. Remove the burgers and set aside.

4. In the skillet, crack the eggs and cook for about 3 minutes, until set.

5. In a small bowl, toss the spinach and grape tomatoes with the remaining 1 tablespoon of olive oil, and season with salt and pepper. Divide the spinach and tomatoes between two plates, top each with a burger, and add an egg on top. Season with salt and pepper.

Variation: Sliced black olives are also a great flavor addition to the salad.

MACRONUTRIENTS	71% FAT	24% PROTEIN	5% CARBS

CALORIES: 531; TOTAL FAT: 42G; PROTEIN: 33G; TOTAL CARBS: 7G; FIBER: 3G; NET CARBS: 4G

GARLIC, MUSHROOM, AND BACON BURGER

PREP TIME: 5 MINUTES **COOK TIME:** 15 MINUTES

I love mushrooms; my daughter does not. But if I mix enough bacon into them and put them on top of a thick, juicy burger, then she can be convinced to eat them, since there are some great rich, savory flavors in this dish. *Serves 2*

- ● ALLERGEN-FREE
- ○ COMFORT FOOD
- ◔ DAIRY-FREE
- ● NUT-FREE
- ● PALEO OR PALEO-FRIENDLY
- ○ SUPER QUICK

4 bacon slices, cut into 1-inch pieces

2 cups sliced mushrooms

1 garlic clove, minced

1 shallot, thinly sliced

Salt

Freshly ground black pepper

½ pound ground beef

1 tablespoon extra-virgin olive oil

1. In a large skillet, cook the bacon over medium-high heat for about 6 minutes, until cooked but not crispy. Add the mushrooms and cook for 6 more minutes. Add the garlic and shallot to the skillet and cook for 2 more minutes. Season with salt and pepper.

2. While the bacon is cooking, create two burger patties and season with salt and pepper.

3. In another large skillet, heat the olive oil over medium heat and add the burger patties. Cook each side for 4 to 5 minutes, flipping once.

4. Pour the bacon-mushroom mixture over each burger and serve.

Variation: You can also melt cheese over each burger if you prefer. Gruyère or Swiss both work nicely.

MACRONUTRIENTS	65% FAT	31% PROTEIN	4% CARBS

CALORIES: 382; TOTAL FAT: 28G; PROTEIN: 30G; TOTAL CARBS: 4G; FIBER: 1G; NET CARBS: 3G

SANTA FE GREEN CHILE BURGER

PREP TIME: 20 MINUTES **COOK TIME:** 25 MINUTES

Living in Santa Fe made me appreciate the incredible flavor roasted green chiles can add to just about anything. Seriously, in New Mexico EVERYTHING has green chiles on it! In this recipe, I roast the green chiles under the broiler because I don't trust myself with open flames. The charring and peeling process of the green chiles takes some time, but the flavor is worth it! *Serves 2*

○ COMFORT FOOD
● NUT-FREE
● PALEO OR PALEO-FRIENDLY

2 Hatch chiles or other green chiles

½ pound ground beef

2 teaspoons chili powder

Salt

Freshly ground black pepper

1 tablespoon extra-virgin olive oil

2 slices pepper jack cheese (optional)

Make It Paleo: You can skip the cheese and instead add a dollop of avocado mayonnaise for a creamy element or Dairy-Free Sour Cream (page 259). Additionally, if you are in a rush, you can use canned green chiles and skip the broiling step altogether.

1. Turn the oven to broil and place a rack in the closest position to it.

2. Line a baking sheet with aluminum foil or a silicone baking mat.

3. Broil the chiles for 10 to 15 minutes, flipping a few times, until they are completely charred on the outside.

4. Transfer the chiles into a resealable bag and let cool for 15 minutes. They will steam in the bag, which will release the charred skin so you can easily peel them.

5. While the chiles are cooling, in a medium bowl, mix the ground beef and chili powder, and season with salt and pepper. Form into two patties.

6. Remove the chiles from the bag and peel off the charred skin. Remove the stem and seeds from the chiles and roughly chop them.

7. In a large skillet, heat the olive oil over medium heat. Add the burger patties and cook on each side for 4 to 5 minutes, flipping once.

8. Cover each cooked burger with half the chiles and top with a slice of cheese. Put a lid on the skillet to melt the cheese and serve.

MACRONUTRIENTS	66% FAT	29% PROTEIN	5% CARBS

CALORIES: 413; TOTAL FAT: 31G; PROTEIN: 30G; TOTAL CARBS: 6G; FIBER: 2G; NET CARBS: 4G

BACON-WRAPPED BURGER

PREP TIME: 15 MINUTES **COOK TIME:** 10 MINUTES

When you wrap a cheeseburger in crispy bacon, only good things can happen. This is a super-simple yet impressive way to make a cheeseburger. I use pepper jack cheese, but you can use whatever variety you have on hand. *Serves 2*

○ COMFORT FOOD
● NUT-FREE
○ SUPER QUICK

½ pound ground beef

Salt

Freshly ground black pepper

8 bacon slices

2 slices pepper jack cheese

1 tablespoon olive oil

1. In a medium bowl, season the ground beef with salt and pepper and divide into four thin patties. Sandwich each cheese slice between two patties and pinch the edges all the way around until the cheese is sealed inside.

2. Basket weave 4 bacon slices and then wrap them around a burger patty. To do that, place 2 slices of bacon vertically on a plate very close to each other, then place 2 slices horizontally. Weave the slices over and then under. It should look like a flat, woven sheet of bacon.

3. Repeat for the other burger.

4. In a skillet, heat the olive oil over medium heat. Cook the burgers for 4 to 5 minutes on each side, flipping once, until the bacon is crispy. Using tongs, turn the burgers onto their sides to crisp the bacon.

Make It Paleo: You can replace the cheese with the dairy-free variety or stuff the burgers with avocado instead.

MACRONUTRIENTS	65% FAT	34% PROTEIN	1% CARBS

CALORIES: 562; TOTAL FAT: 40G; PROTEIN: 46G; TOTAL CARBS: 2G; FIBER: 0G; NET CARBS: 2G

"SPAGHETTI" AND MEAT SAUCE

PREP TIME: 5 MINUTES COOK TIME: 8 HOURS

Slow cooker meat sauce is a beautiful thing! Just let it cook all day long, and then dinner comes together in minutes—whether you choose Zoodles (zucchini noodles, page 37) or Shirataki Noodles (page 40) to smother with the rich, meaty sauce. The carbs in tomatoes can add up, so this sauce is heavier on the meat and lighter on the tomatoes than a traditional sauce. *Serves 2*

- ● ALLERGEN-FREE
- ○ COMFORT FOOD
- ◐ DAIRY-FREE
- ● NUT-FREE
- ● PALEO OR PALEO-FRIENDLY

1 tablespoon extra-virgin olive oil

¼ pound ground Italian sausage, not in casing

¼ pound ground beef

1 shallot, minced

1 garlic clove, minced

½ cup low-sugar marinara sauce

¼ cup beef broth or beef bone broth

1 tablespoon Italian Seasoning (page 246)

1 batch Zoodles (page 37) or 1 batch Shirataki Noodles (page 40)

1. Preheat the slow cooker on low.

2. In a skillet, heat the olive oil over medium-high heat. Add the Italian sausage and ground beef and cook for 6 minutes, until browned.

3. Add the shallot and garlic and stir well. Cook for 2 more minutes.

4. Transfer the meat mixture to the slow cooker and top with the marinara sauce, beef broth, and Italian seasoning.

5. Cover and cook for 8 hours.

6. Top the noodles with the meat sauce and serve.

Variation: If you eat dairy, you can add a splash of heavy whipping cream to the slow cooker for the last 10 minutes of cooking. I like how the cream brings out the richness of the flavors.

MACRONUTRIENTS	71% FAT	19% PROTEIN	10% CARBS

CALORIES: 495; TOTAL FAT: 39G; PROTEIN: 24G; TOTAL CARBS: 11G; FIBER: 3G; NET CARBS: 8G

GREEN CHILE MEATBALLS

PREP TIME: 10 MINUTES **COOK TIME:** 30 MINUTES

A fun southwestern take on traditional meatballs, these feature taco seasoning and use crushed pork rinds as a replacement for bread crumbs to hold them together. *Serves 2*

○ COMFORT FOOD

◔ DAIRY-FREE

● NUT-FREE

● PALEO OR PALEO-FRIENDLY

¼ pound ground pork

¼ pound ground beef

¼ cup canned green chiles

¼ cup Pork Rind "Bread" Crumbs (page 249)

1 large egg

2 teaspoons Taco Seasoning (page 245)

½ cup salsa verde

1. Preheat the oven to 400°F.

2. In a bowl, mix the pork, beef, green chiles, pork rinds, egg, and taco seasoning.

3. Form the mixture into 8 meatballs and place in a baking dish.

4. Pour the salsa verde over the meatballs.

5. Cover the dish with aluminum foil.

6. Bake for 30 minutes, uncovering the dish for the last 5 minutes.

Variation: I like to mix ground beef and pork for these, but they work just as well with just ground beef or just ground pork. If you want to use fresh green chiles, see the roasting instructions in the Santa Fe Green Chile Burger (page 195) recipe.

MACRONUTRIENTS	61% FAT	32% PROTEIN	7% CARBS

CALORIES: 326; TOTAL FAT: 22G; PROTEIN: 26G; TOTAL CARBS: 6G; FIBER: 1G; NET CARBS: 5G

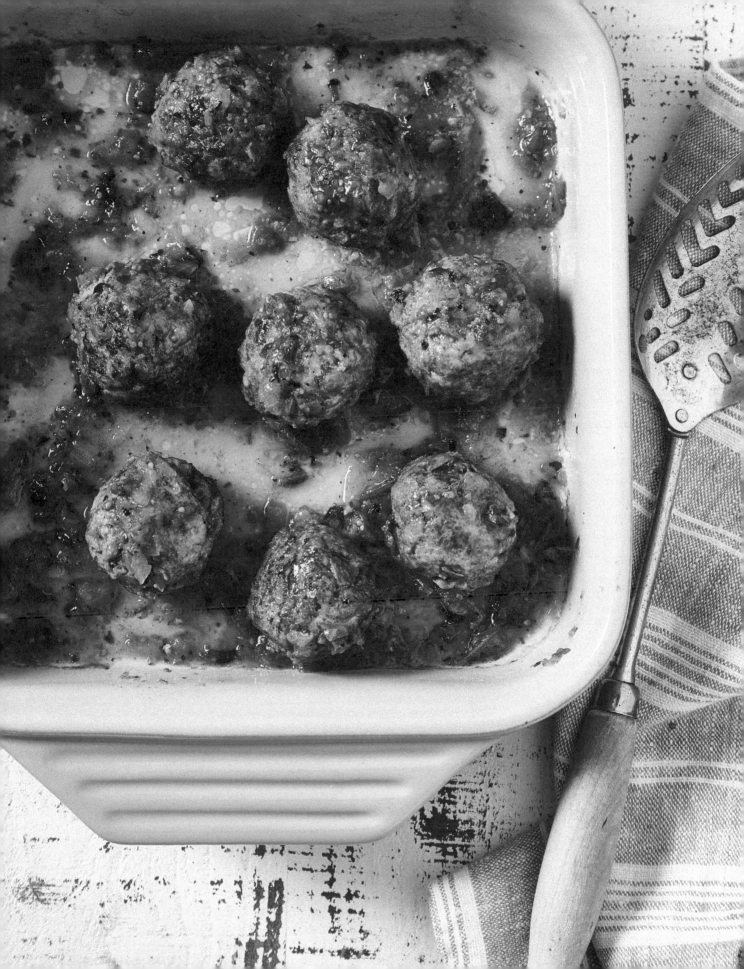

BACON-WRAPPED STEAK BITES
WITH MUSTARD DIPPING SAUCE

PREP TIME: 10 MINUTES **COOK TIME:** 10 MINUTES

The Oven-Baked Garlic and Herb Steak (page 190), which is made in foil packets, is one great option for cubes of steak, otherwise known as beef tips, and this recipe is another. Beef tips are usually affordably priced, and they are great for dipping and wrapping in bacon. *Serves 2*

- ALLERGEN-FREE
- COMFORT FOOD
- DAIRY-FREE
- NUT-FREE
- PALEO OR PALEO-FRIENDLY
- SUPER QUICK

4 bacon slices, halved crosswise

8 ounces sirloin steak, cut into 2-inch cubes

1 tablespoon extra-virgin olive oil

2 tablespoons avocado oil mayonnaise

1 tablespoon Dijon mustard

1 teaspoon vinegar

¼ teaspoon garlic powder

Salt

Freshly ground black pepper

1. Wrap half a slice of bacon around each piece of steak. Secure with a toothpick.

2. In a skillet, heat the olive oil over medium-high heat.

3. Add the beef pieces and sear on each beef side for 1 minute.

4. Turn the beef pieces onto one bacon side and cook 2 minutes, then flip and put the other bacon side down for 2 more minutes, until the bacon reaches your desired crispiness.

5. Remove the beef pieces from the pan and arrange on a serving plate.

6. In a small bowl, combine the mayonnaise, Dijon, vinegar, and garlic powder. Season with salt and pepper.

Variation: Creamy horseradish also pairs really well with this dish.

MACRONUTRIENTS	66% FAT	30% PROTEIN	4% CARBS

CALORIES: 419; TOTAL FAT: 31G; PROTEIN: 30G; TOTAL CARBS: 4G; FIBER: 0G; NET CARBS: 4G

MINI MEATLOAF

PREP TIME: 10 MINUTES **COOK TIME:** 35 MINUTES

Meatloaf is definitely a comfort food. I use my mini loaf pans to make
these into single-serving meatloafs, but you can use a muffin tin instead.
This recipe is an easy one to reheat for quick lunches. *Serves 2*

- ● ALLERGEN-FREE
- ○ COMFORT FOOD
- ● DAIRY-FREE
- ● NUT-FREE
- ● PALEO OR PALEO-FRIENDLY

Butter, ghee, oil, or nonstick
cooking spray, for greasing

¼ pound ground Italian sausage,
not in casing

¼ pound ground beef

½ cup diced mushrooms

1 shallot, diced

1 garlic clove, minced

1 tablespoon Italian Seasoning
(page 246)

Salt

Freshly ground black pepper

4 bacon slices

1. Preheat the oven to 400°F.

2. Grease a mini loaf pan or muffin tin with butter.

3. In a medium bowl, combine the sausage, ground
   beef, mushrooms, shallot, garlic, and Italian
   seasoning. Season with salt and pepper. Using
   your hands, mix well.

4. Divide in half for mini loaf pans or into quarters
   for muffin tins, and form into mini loaves.

5. Wrap 2 slices of bacon around each mini meatloaf and secure with a toothpick.

6. Bake for 35 minutes.

7. Let cool for 10 minutes and then serve.

Make Ahead: To reheat, just cover with aluminum foil
and heat in the oven.

MACRONUTRIENTS	71% FAT	26% PROTEIN	3% CARBS

CALORIES: 398; TOTAL FAT: 31G; PROTEIN: 26G; TOTAL CARBS: 3G; FIBER: 0G; NET CARBS: 3G

KETO CHICKEN-FRIED STEAK

PREP TIME: 15 MINUTES **COOK TIME:** 10 MINUTES

Crispy chicken-fried steak gets a keto makeover with ground pork rinds and coconut flour. Make sure you get the oil nice and hot before adding the dredged steak—you want it to really sizzle so it gets perfectly crispy. *Serves 2*

○ COMFORT FOOD
◐ DAIRY-FREE
● NUT-FREE
● PALEO OR PALEO-FRIENDLY
○ SUPER QUICK

½ pound cube steak

1 large egg

½ cup coconut flour

1 teaspoon cayenne pepper

Salt

Freshly ground black pepper

½ cup Pork Rind "Bread" Crumbs (page 249)*

¼ cup extra-virgin olive oil, or enough to coat the bottom of the skillet

1. Using a mallet, pound the cube steak to tenderize it.

2. In a shallow bowl, lightly beat the egg. On a large plate, mix the coconut flour and cayenne pepper. Season with salt and pepper. On another large plate, add the pork rind "bread" crumbs.

3. Dredge the steak on both sides in the coconut flour mixture. Dip into the egg, coating both sides. Dredge in the pork rind crumbs, pressing the pork rinds into the steak so they stick.

4. In a large skillet, heat the olive oil over medium-high heat until the oil sizzles. Cook the "breaded" steak for 4 minutes per side, flipping once, until golden and crispy.

Variation: You can add additional seasoning to the "breading" by using flavored pork rinds or adding Taco Seasoning (page 245).

*Note: The macros will be slightly different if you have leftover "breading mix" and/or oil in the skillet. These numbers include all of the "breading" and oil.

MACRONUTRIENTS	36% FAT	41% PROTEIN	23% CARBS

CALORIES: 485; TOTAL FAT: 30G; PROTEIN: 34G; TOTAL CARBS: 19G; FIBER: 12G; NET CARBS: 7G

CHEESEBURGER TACOS

PREP TIME: 10 MINUTES **COOK TIME:** 20 MINUTES

This recipe packs in all the familiar flavors of a cheeseburger inside a crunchy taco shell made out of cheese! Kids will love this dish, and it will turn your taco Tuesdays keto. Anything you like on a burger can be added! *Serves 2*

○ COMFORT FOOD
● NUT-FREE
○ SUPER QUICK

1 tablespoon extra-virgin olive oil

¼ pound ground beef

¼ onion, diced

Salt

Freshly ground black pepper

2 cups shredded cheese

¼ cup shredded lettuce

1 tablespoon avocado oil mayonnaise

1 tablespoon yellow mustard

¼ cup pickle slices

1. Preheat the oven to 350°F. Line a baking sheet with parchment paper or a silicone baking mat.

2. In a large skillet, heat the olive oil over medium-high heat. Add the ground beef and onion, and season with salt and pepper. Cook for 6 minutes, stirring regularly, until fully cooked.

3. Place ½-cup mounds of cheese on the prepared baking sheet. Bake the large "cheese chips" for about 7 minutes, or until the edges are brown and the middle has melted.

4. While the cheese chips are baking, set two drinking glasses upside down, with a thick kitchen spoon or spatula balanced on top of them.

5. Remove the baking sheet from the oven. Using a spatula, place each cheese chip over the kitchen spoon or spatula and let it hang and crisp up in a taco shell shape. You will need to move quickly to get each cheese chip folded before it fully hardens. Then let the shells harden for 5 minutes before filling them.

6. Stuff the cheese shells with the beef, shredded lettuce, mayonnaise, mustard, and pickle slices.

Variation: Crumbled bacon and sliced avocado also make great additions.

MACRONUTRIENTS	72% FAT	25% PROTEIN	3% CARBS

CALORIES: 663; TOTAL FAT: 54G; PROTEIN: 40G; TOTAL CARBS: 5G; FIBER: 1G; NET CARBS: 4G

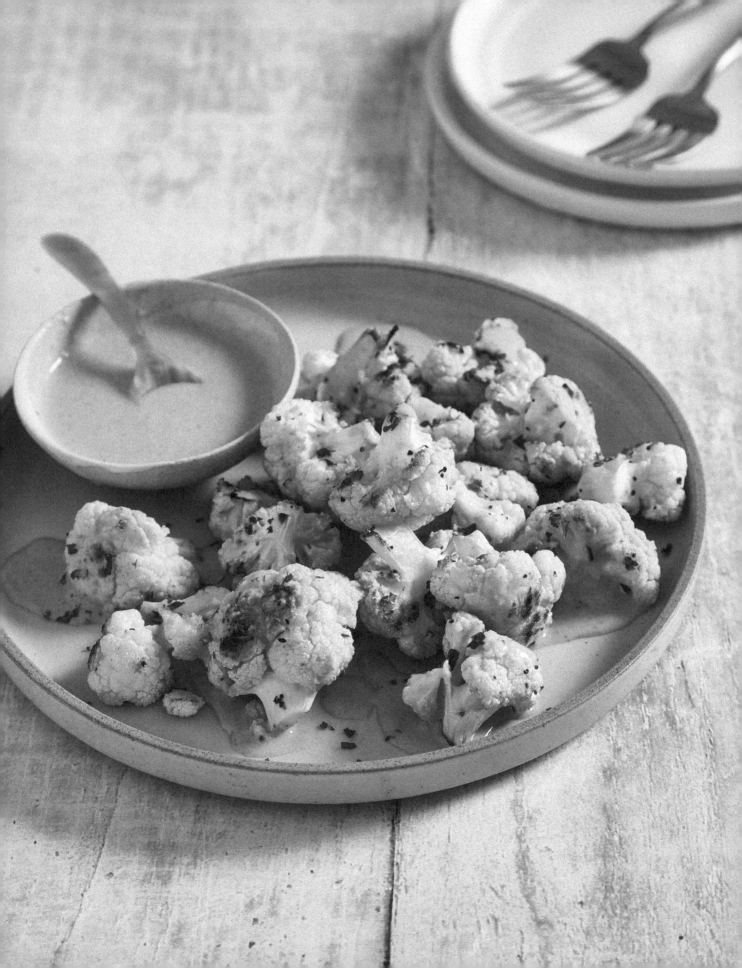

SIDES

CHAPTER TWELVE

Opposite: Thai Peanut Roasted Cauliflower

CUCUMBER BITES

PREP TIME: 10 MINUTES

Cucumbers are a great vehicle for flavors. For these I like to create what are basically cucumber shot glasses. Sounds fun, right? It is! Fill them up with dairy-free cream cheese and any other flavor combinations you can dream up. *Serves 2*

○ COMFORT FOOD

◐ DAIRY-FREE

● PALEO OR PALEO-FRIENDLY

○ SUPER QUICK

1 cucumber

Salt

2 tablespoons Dairy-Free Cream Cheese (page 258)

1 cooked bacon slice, crumbled

½ jalapeño pepper, diced fine

1. Cut the cucumber into 1-inch slices and scoop the seeds out of the top to create a cup (or shot glass as I like to call it). I peel my cucumber, but you don't have to. Season with salt.

2. In a small bowl, mix the dairy-free cream cheese with the crumbled bacon and jalapeño pepper. Spoon the mixture into the cucumber cups.

Variation: Dill and little bits of smoked salmon is another yummy combination. You can also use the Dairy-Free Avocado Crema (page 257) paired with the Chili-Lime Seasoning (page 244).

MACRONUTRIENTS	64% FAT	13% PROTEIN	23% CARBS

CALORIES: 95; TOTAL FAT: 7G; PROTEIN: 3G; TOTAL CARBS: 6G; FIBER: 1G; NET CARBS: 5G

CRISPY BRUSSELS SPROUT LEAVES

PREP TIME: 10 MINUTES **COOK TIME:** 12 MINUTES

A restaurant near my office serves up crispy Brussels sprout leaves, and I love how light they are compared to the entire sprout. There's a bit of prep work separating the leaves from the core, but it's worth it! To prepare, just peel the individual leaves off the sprouts and discard the thick core. *Serves 2*

⬤ ALLERGEN-FREE
◯ COMFORT FOOD
◗ DAIRY-FREE
⬤ NUT-FREE
⬤ PALEO OR PALEO-FRIENDLY
◯ SUPER QUICK

1 cup Brussels sprout leaves

½ tablespoon extra-virgin olive oil

2 teaspoons lemon zest

Salt

Freshly ground black pepper

1. Preheat the oven to 375°F. Line a baking sheet with parchment paper or a silicone baking mat.

2. In a mixing bowl, toss the Brussels sprout leaves with olive oil and lemon zest. Season with salt and pepper.

3. Roast for 12 minutes, until the leaves are crispy.

Variation: I like to add flakes of Parmesan and toasted hazelnuts to mine.

MACRONUTRIENTS	63% FAT	7% PROTEIN	30% CARBS

CALORIES: 49; TOTAL FAT: 4G; PROTEIN: 1G; TOTAL CARBS: 4G; FIBER: 2G; NET CARBS: 2G

BAKED PARMESAN TOMATOES

PREP TIME: 5 MINUTES **COOK TIME:** 10 MINUTES

Think of this as a baked version of a caprese salad—tomatoes, Parmesan, and basil served up in a warm, melty way that you will love. *Serves 2*

○ COMFORT FOOD

● NUT-FREE

○ SUPER QUICK

1 large tomato, cut into 4 slices

1 teaspoon Italian Seasoning (page 246)

½ cup shaved Parmesan

1 teaspoon sliced fresh basil

1. Preheat the oven to 400°F. Line a baking sheet with parchment paper or a silicone baking mat.

2. On the prepared baking sheet, arrange the tomatoes in a single layer. Sprinkle with the Italian seasoning and top with the Parmesan and basil.

3. Bake until the cheese is bubbling, about 10 minutes.

Variation: You can do a Mexican take on this recipe using Chili-Lime Seasoning (page 244) or Taco Seasoning (page 245), Oaxaca cheese, and a slice of jalapeño pepper on top.

MACRONUTRIENTS	52% FAT	35% PROTEIN	13% CARBS

CALORIES: 124; TOTAL FAT: 7G; PROTEIN: 10G; TOTAL CARBS: 5G; FIBER: 1G; NET CARBS: 4G

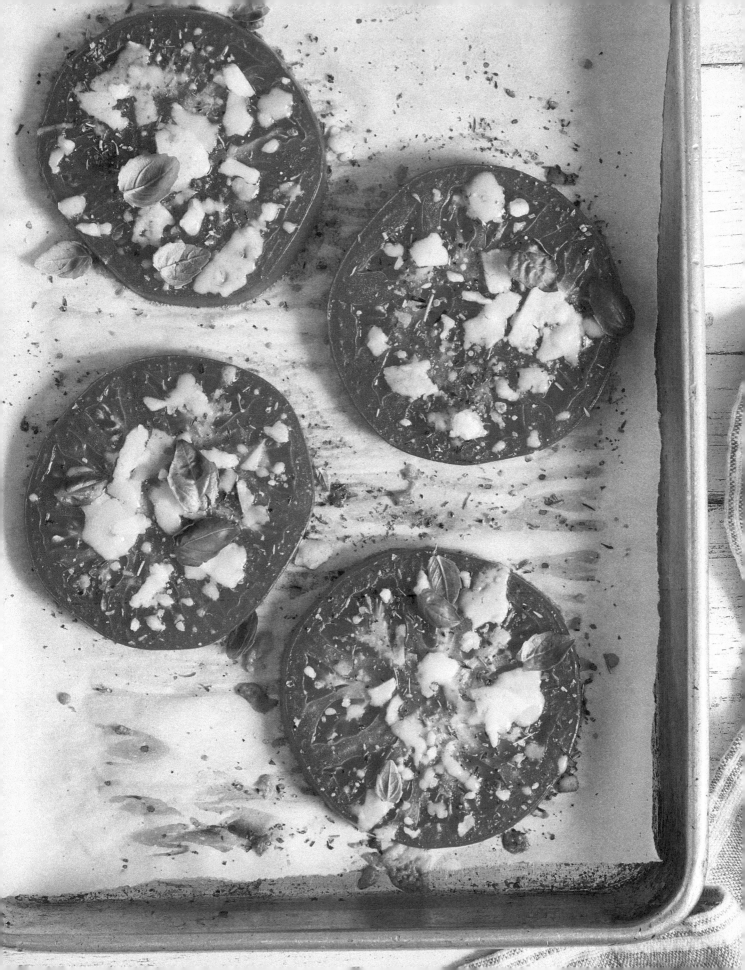

LEMONY SPINACH

PREP TIME: 5 MINUTES **COOK TIME:** 5 MINUTES

If you are looking for a light and fresh side dish that can be ready in minutes, this is the perfect choice. Lemon and spinach get the top billing, but in my opinion the capers steal the show! *Serves 2*

● ALLERGEN-FREE
○ COMFORT FOOD
◐ DAIRY-FREE
● NUT-FREE
● PALEO OR PALEO-FRIENDLY
○ SUPER QUICK

1 tablespoon extra-virgin olive oil or ghee

1 garlic clove, minced

1 shallot, thinly sliced

4 cups fresh spinach

¼ lemon, juiced

1 tablespoon capers, chopped

Salt

Freshly ground black pepper

1. In a skillet, heat the olive oil over medium heat. Add the garlic and the shallot, and sauté for 1 minute, stirring continuously.

2. Add the whole-leaf spinach, lemon juice, and capers. Cook for 1 minute, until the spinach is just wilted. Season with salt and pepper.

3. Divide between two plates and top with the lemon zest.

| MACRONUTRIENTS | 76% FAT | 6% PROTEIN | 18% CARBS |

CALORIES: 82; TOTAL FAT: 7G; PROTEIN: 2G; TOTAL CARBS: 4G; FIBER: 2G; NET CARBS: 2G

CHEESY ROASTED ASPARAGUS

PREP TIME: 10 MINUTES **COOK TIME:** 10 MINUTES

Asparagus has always been my go-to vegetable throughout my adult life. In my opinion, roasted is the best way to eat asparagus, especially when it is covered in Parmesan cheese! *Serves 2*

○ COMFORT FOOD
● NUT-FREE
○ SUPER QUICK

1 bunch asparagus

2 tablespoons extra-virgin olive oil

¼ cup Pork Rind "Bread" Crumbs (page 249) (optional)

½ cup grated Parmesan cheese

½ teaspoon garlic powder

Salt

Freshly ground black pepper

1. Preheat the oven to 425°F.

2. Snap the woody ends off the asparagus, wherever they naturally snap off.

3. In a large plastic ziptop bag, combine the asparagus and olive oil and shake. Open the bag and add the ground pork rinds (if using), Parmesan cheese, and garlic powder. Season with salt and pepper. Shake until fully coated.

4. On a baking sheet, arrange the asparagus in a single layer and roast for 8 to 10 minutes.

Variation: If you like the extra kick of garlic, you can top the coated asparagus with 2 cloves of minced fresh garlic just before roasting.

MACRONUTRIENTS	73% FAT	19% PROTEIN	8% CARBS

CALORIES: 253; TOTAL FAT: 21G; PROTEIN: 12G; TOTAL CARBS: 6G; FIBER: 3G; NET CARBS: 3G

ROASTED GARLIC BROCCOLI WITH ALMONDS

PREP TIME: 5 MINUTES **COOK TIME:** 25 MINUTES

I never liked broccoli as a kid, probably because my mom never roasted it! I'm convinced that roasting is the key to making any vegetable delicious. This recipe has all kinds of amazing flavors mixed in, but the garlic and sliced almonds are my favorite parts! *Serves 2*

○ COMFORT FOOD

½ broccoli head, cut into bite-size florets

2 tablespoons extra-virgin olive oil or ghee

1 teaspoon red pepper flakes

1 garlic clove, minced

Salt

2 tablespoons sliced almonds

2 lemon wedges

2 tablespoons grated Parmesan cheese

1. Preheat the oven to 400°F. Line a baking sheet with parchment paper or a silicone baking mat.

2. In a bowl, toss the broccoli with the olive oil, red pepper flakes, and garlic. Season with salt.

3. On the prepared baking sheet, arrange the broccoli in a single layer and roast for 20 minutes.

4. Stir the broccoli, add the sliced almonds, and cook for 5 more minutes.

5. Squeeze the lemon wedges over the top and sprinkle the Parmesan cheese all over.

Make It Paleo: You can omit the Parmesan cheese, and this broccoli will still be amazing.

MACRONUTRIENTS	68% FAT	13% PROTEIN	19% CARBS

CALORIES: 251; TOTAL FAT: 19G; PROTEIN: 8G; TOTAL CARBS: 12G; FIBER: 5G; NET CARBS: 7G

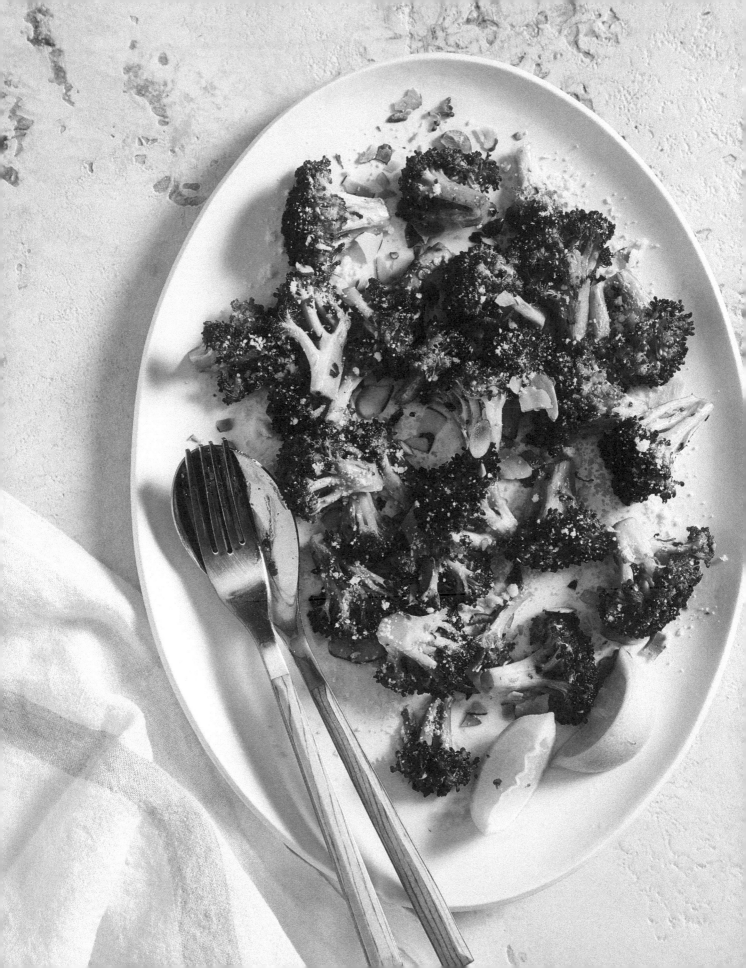

BUFFALO CAULIFLOWER

PREP TIME: 5 MINUTES   COOK TIME: 30 MINUTES

A vegetarian version of buffalo wings for the win! These are delicious, vegetarian or not. Dip them in creamy blue cheese dressing or just eat them plain. *Serves 2*

● ALLERGEN-FREE
○ COMFORT FOOD
◔ DAIRY-FREE
● NUT-FREE
● PALEO OR PALEO-FRIENDLY

½ cauliflower head, cut into florets

1 tablespoon extra-virgin olive oil

1 teaspoon garlic powder

Salt

Freshly ground black pepper

1 tablespoon butter or ghee

¼ cup buffalo wing sauce

1. Preheat the oven to 400°F. Line a baking sheet with parchment paper or a silicone baking mat.

2. In a mixing bowl, drizzle the cauliflower with olive oil and add the garlic powder. Season with salt and pepper and toss well.

3. On a baking sheet, arrange the cauliflower in a single layer and roast for 15 minutes. Flip the cauliflower and continue to cook for 10 more minutes.

4. In a small saucepan, mix the butter and buffalo wing sauce over medium heat until melted and combined.

5. Brush the cauliflower with the sauce and cook for 5 more minutes. Serve.

Variation: These cauliflower bites pair nicely with the Dairy-Free Sour Cream (page 259) as a dipping sauce.

MACRONUTRIENTS	80% FAT	6% PROTEIN	14% CARBS

CALORIES: 145; TOTAL FAT: 13G; PROTEIN: 2G; TOTAL CARBS: 5G; FIBER: 2G; NET CARBS: 3G

ROASTED CAULIFLOWER WITH BACON

PREP TIME: 5 MINUTES **COOK TIME:** 30 MINUTES

Two of my favorite keto ingredients are cauliflower and bacon, so it's only natural to combine them. I could eat this every day, and I am guessing you will feel the same way. You can add so many other things to this bacon and cauliflower combination. I love adding capers or sliced pepperoncini. *Serves 2*

- ● ALLERGEN-FREE
- ○ COMFORT FOOD
- ◐ DAIRY-FREE
- ● NUT-FREE
- ● PALEO OR PALEO-FRIENDLY

½ cauliflower head, cut into bite-size florets

4 bacon slices, cut into bite-size pieces

1 tablespoon extra-virgin olive oil

Salt

Freshly ground black pepper

1. Preheat the oven to 400°F. Line a baking sheet with parchment paper or a silicone baking mat.

2. On the prepared baking sheet, arrange the cauliflower and bacon in a single layer. Drizzle with the olive oil and season with salt and pepper. Don't add too much salt, because the bacon grease will coat the cauliflower as it cooks.

3. Roast for 25 to 30 minutes, stirring once halfway through, until the bacon is crispy and the cauliflower is tender and browned.

MACRONUTRIENTS	82% FAT	10% PROTEIN	8% CARBS

CALORIES: 352; TOTAL FAT: 32G; PROTEIN: 9G; TOTAL CARBS: 8G; FIBER: 4G; NET CARBS: 4G

THAI PEANUT ROASTED CAULIFLOWER

PREP TIME: 10 MINUTES **COOK TIME:** 20 MINUTES

I absolutely love peanut sauce! I know peanut butter is one of those controversial keto foods since peanuts are a legume, but I love to use a low-sugar peanut butter periodically. This is another side dish that I often eat as my meal. *Serves 2*

○ COMFORT FOOD
◑ DAIRY-FREE
○ SUPER QUICK

½ cauliflower head, cut into bite-size florets

1 tablespoon extra-virgin olive oil

Salt

Freshly ground black pepper

½ cup unsweetened full-fat coconut milk

2 tablespoons peanut butter

¼ teaspoon red curry paste

1 garlic clove, minced

1 tablespoon chopped fresh parsley or dried

1. Preheat the oven to 400°F.

2. On a baking sheet, arrange the cauliflower in a single layer. Drizzle with the olive oil and season with salt and pepper. Roast for about 20 minutes, until the edges are brown.

3. While the cauliflower is cooking, in a blender, combine the coconut milk, peanut butter, curry paste, and garlic. Process until smooth.

4. Once the cauliflower is finished, divide it between two plates and drizzle the peanut sauce on top. Garnish with the parsley.

Make It Paleo: Replace the peanut butter with a paleo-approved nut butter.

MACRONUTRIENTS	80% FAT	9% PROTEIN	11% CARBS

CALORIES: 290; TOTAL FAT: 27G; PROTEIN: 8G; TOTAL CARBS: 9G; FIBER: 3G; NET CARBS: 6G

CRAB-STUFFED MUSHROOMS

PREP TIME: 10 MINUTES **COOK TIME:** 15 MINUTES

You might feel a little fancy when you make these; I know I do. They are the perfect little restaurant bite, but super easy to make. These are a great side dish, meal, or appetizer for a party. *Serves 2*

○ COMFORT FOOD
◐ DAIRY-FREE
● NUT-FREE
● PALEO OR PALEO-FRIENDLY
○ SUPER QUICK

2 ounces lump crab meat

2 tablespoons avocado oil mayonnaise

1 tablespoon sliced scallions, green parts only

¼ teaspoon paprika

¼ teaspoon onion powder

Salt

Freshly ground black pepper

6 to 8 cremini mushrooms, stemmed

1 teaspoon chopped fresh parsley or dried

1. Preheat the oven to 350°F. Line a baking sheet with parchment paper or a silicone mat.

2. In a medium bowl, mix the crab meat, mayonnaise, scallions, paprika, and onion powder. Season with salt and pepper.

3. On the prepared baking sheet, arrange the mushrooms, gill side up, and fill each with a spoonful of the crab mixture.

4. Bake for 15 minutes.

5. Garnish with the parsley to serve.

Variation: You can also make this with salmon if you don't have lump crab.

MACRONUTRIENTS	65% FAT	23% PROTEIN	12% CARBS

CALORIES: 139; TOTAL FAT: 10G; PROTEIN: 8G; TOTAL CARBS: 3G; FIBER: 1G; NET CARBS: 2G

BUFFALO "WING" DEVILED EGGS

PREP TIME: 15 MINUTES **COOK TIME:** 15 MINUTES

Note the serving size on this recipe, because who eats just one deviled egg? Definitely not me! These are fun because you bring in the flavors of buffalo wings with a touch of blue cheese, perfect for a football day. *Serves 6*

○ COMFORT FOOD
● NUT-FREE
○ SUPER QUICK

6 large eggs

¼ cup avocado oil mayonnaise

2 tablespoons sour cream

2 tablespoons buffalo wing sauce

2 teaspoons ground mustard

Salt

Freshly ground black pepper

¼ cup blue cheese crumbles

1 tablespoon chopped fresh chives

1. In a saucepan, cover the eggs with water. Place over high heat, and bring the water to a boil. Once it is boiling, turn off the heat, cover, and leave on the burner for 10 to 12 minutes. Submerge the cooked eggs in a bowl of ice-cold water to stop the cooking and then peel off the shells.

2. Halve the eggs lengthwise. With a small spoon, carefully remove the yolks, reserving the whites on a plate. Transfer the yolks to a small bowl and mash them.

3. Add the mayonnaise, sour cream, buffalo wing sauce, and mustard. Season with salt and pepper. Mix with a fork until smooth.

4. Arrange the egg whites on a plate with the cut sides facing up. Spoon or pipe the yolk mixture back into the egg white cavities. I pipe them with a small bag with the corner cut off. Sprinkle the blue cheese crumbles and chives over the top.

Make Ahead: You can store these covered in the refrigerator for a few days.

MACRONUTRIENTS	77% FAT	20% PROTEIN	3% CARBS

CALORIES: 223; TOTAL FAT: 19G PROTEIN: 11G; TOTAL CARBS: 2G; FIBER: 1G; NET CARBS: 1G

SAVORY CHEDDAR AND CHIVE WAFFLES

PREP TIME: 10 MINUTES **COOK TIME:** 10 MINUTES

I like to experiment in the kitchen, and recently I wondered what would happen if I put my keto bread batter together and cooked it in my waffle iron instead of baking it in the oven. Turns out, it works perfectly! To take it a step further, I added Cheddar and chives to the original recipe to create what I think is the perfect side dish when you just want to slather some butter on yummy bread! *Serves 6*

○ **COMFORT FOOD**
○ **SUPER QUICK**

5 tablespoons butter, at room temperature

6 large eggs

1½ cups almond flour

3 teaspoons baking powder

Salt

¾ cup shredded Cheddar cheese

¼ cup chopped fresh chives

1. Preheat the waffle iron.

2. In a mixing bowl, combine the butter, eggs, almond flour, and baking powder. Season with salt. Using a hand or stand mixer, thoroughly mix the ingredients at medium speed. Be sure to scrape the mixing bowl to get everything incorporated.

3. Fold in the cheese and chives by hand.

4. Grease the waffle iron and pour in ¼ to ½ cup of batter, depending on your waffle iron, making sure not to overfill.

5. Cook according to the waffle iron settings (mine beeps when it is done). The waffles should be golden and crispy. Remove the savory waffle and repeat. There are so many different-size waffle irons that it is hard to say exactly how many the recipe will make for you, but it makes 6 (4-inch) waffles for me.

Variation: The possibilities are endless with these. Fold crumbled bacon in the batter or diced jalapeño peppers—go crazy!

MACRONUTRIENTS	74% FAT	18% PROTEIN	8% CARBS

CALORIES: 364; TOTAL FAT: 30G; PROTEIN: 16G; TOTAL CARBS: 7G; FIBER: 3G; NET CARBS: 4G

BACON-WRAPPED ASPARAGUS

PREP TIME: 10 MINUTES **COOK TIME:** 20 MINUTES

Crispy, salty, buttery, and delicious are four words that describe this dish.
I can't imagine anyone not loving these. *Serves 2*

○ COMFORT FOOD
◐ DAIRY-FREE
● NUT-FREE
● PALEO OR PALEO-FRIENDLY
○ SUPER QUICK

2 tablespoons butter or ghee

1 teaspoon soy sauce or
coconut aminos

Pinch freshly ground black pepper

Pinch garlic powder

6 thick asparagus spears

6 bacon slices

1. Preheat the oven to 400°F. Line a baking sheet with parchment paper or a silicone baking mat.

2. In a small saucepan, combine the butter, soy sauce, pepper, and garlic powder and cook over low heat. Continue to simmer to let the sauce thicken while you wrap the bacon around the asparagus.

3. Wrap 1 bacon slice around each spear of asparagus and then place the spears on the baking sheet.

4. Brush the butter mixture onto the bacon and cook for 20 minutes, until the bacon is crispy.

Variation: If you can find only thin asparagus, you can wrap one bacon slice around multiple spears of asparagus.

MACRONUTRIENTS	78% FAT	18% PROTEIN	4% CARBS

CALORIES: 244; TOTAL FAT: 21G; PROTEIN: 11G; TOTAL CARBS: 3G; FIBER: 1G; NET CARBS: 2G

KALE AND BUTTERNUT SQUASH GRATIN

PREP TIME: 10 MINUTES **COOK TIME:** 25 MINUTES

I love this side dish—it is coziness on a plate. I have made this two years in a row for Thanksgiving, and everyone loves it. It's definitely rich, and you don't need a lot—I often just make this side dish my dinner. *Serves 2*

○ COMFORT FOOD
● NUT-FREE

½ cup cubed butternut squash

2 tablespoons extra-virgin olive oil or ghee, divided

Salt

Freshly ground black pepper

1 garlic clove, minced

½ shallot, thinly sliced

1 cup chopped kale

2 tablespoons shredded Gruyère cheese

1 tablespoon heavy whipping cream

¼ cup Pork Rind "Bread" Crumbs (page 249)

1 tablespoon grated Parmesan cheese

1 teaspoon dried oregano

1. Preheat the oven to 425°F. Line a baking sheet with parchment paper or a silicone baking mat.

2. On the prepared baking sheet, arrange the squash in a single layer. Drizzle with 1 tablespoon of olive oil and season with salt and pepper. Roast for 10 minutes.

3. While the squash is roasting, in a medium skillet, heat the remaining 1 tablespoon of olive oil over medium heat.

4. Add the garlic and shallot and cook for about 3 minutes, until softened. Add the kale and cook for 2 more minutes, stirring, until it wilts.

5. Remove the skillet from the heat and add the Gruyère cheese and heavy cream, and stir to combine.

6. Add the roasted butternut squash to the skillet. Season with salt and pepper, and stir to combine.

7. Pour the mixture into a small baking dish.

8. Sprinkle the pork rind crumbs, Parmesan cheese, and oregano on top.

9. Cover loosely with aluminum foil and bake for 10 to 15 minutes, until golden brown. Remove the foil for the last 5 minutes.

Make Ahead: This dish heats up fabulously. I once ate it three nights in a row!

MACRONUTRIENTS	74% FAT	12% PROTEIN	14% CARBS

CALORIES: 266; TOTAL FAT: 22G; PROTEIN: 8G; TOTAL CARBS: 9G; FIBER: 2G; NET CARBS: 7G

SLOW COOKER CAULIFLOWER "FRIED" RICE

PREP TIME: 10 MINUTES **COOK TIME:** 3 HOURS

Cauliflower rice is quick and easy to make. I experimented by throwing it in a slow cooker one day before I went to one of my daughter's volleyball practices and loved the results. Cooking it that way imparted a lot of flavor to the cauliflower rice and made it super tender. *Serves 2*

○ COMFORT FOOD
◔ DAIRY-FREE
● NUT-FREE
● PALEO OR PALEO-FRIENDLY

1 tablespoon sesame oil

½ head cauliflower, riced

¼ cup diced onion

1 tablespoon soy sauce or coconut aminos

¼ cup chicken broth

1 teaspoon garlic powder

1 teaspoon onion powder

¼ teaspoon ground ginger

2 large eggs

¼ cup sliced scallions, green parts only

1. Preheat the slow cooker on low.

2. Drizzle the sesame oil on the bottom of the slow cooker and top with the cauliflower rice, onion, soy sauce, chicken broth, garlic powder, onion powder, and ground ginger.

3. Cover and cook for 2 hours.

4. In a small bowl, beat the eggs, and pour them into the slow cooker. Cover and cook for 1 more hour, stirring occasionally.

5. Divide the cauliflower between two bowls, and top with the scallions to serve.

Variation: Traditionally fried rice includes peas and carrots, but both are higher-carb vegetables, so I leave them out. However, if you would like to add any vegetables, you can do so when you add the eggs.

MACRONUTRIENTS	59% FAT	26% PROTEIN	15% CARBS

CALORIES: 184; TOTAL FAT: 12G; PROTEIN: 10G; TOTAL CARBS: 9G; FIBER: 3G; NET CARBS: 6G

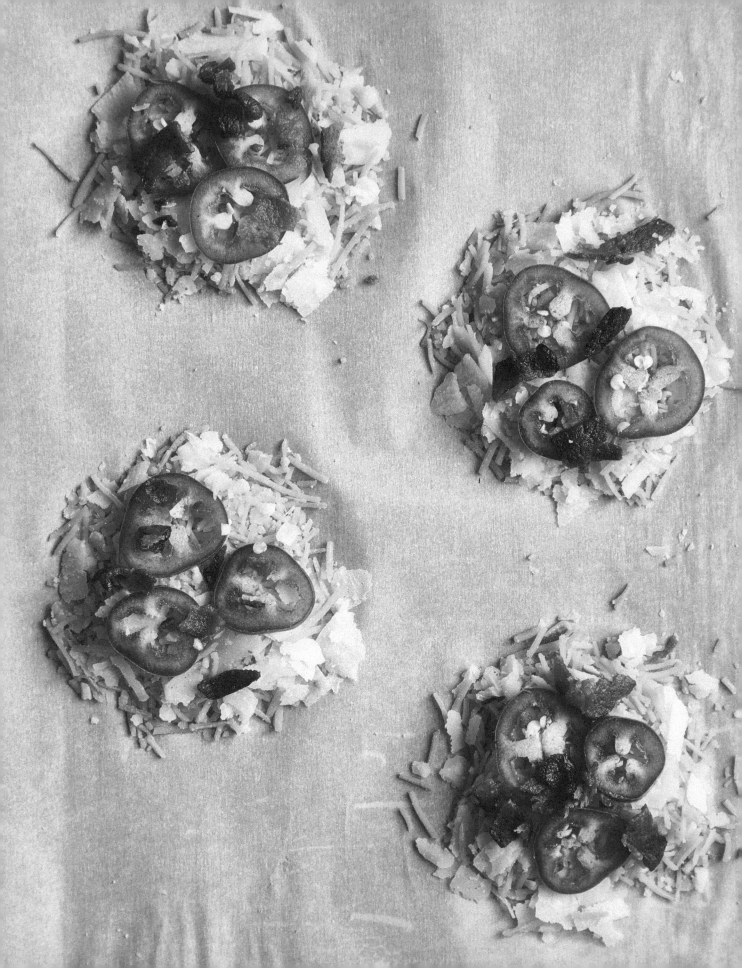

SNACKS

CHAPTER THIRTEEN

Opposite: Bacon Jalapeño Cheese Crisps

PORK RIND CHIPS

PREP TIME: 10 MINUTES **COOK TIME:** 10 MINUTES

Crispy chips to dip are one of the things I missed the most when I started keto. Then I got creative with some pork rinds and cheese, and this recipe was born! There are more flavors of pork rinds available in stores these days, so feel free to experiment with different combinations. *Serves 2*

○ COMFORT FOOD
● NUT-FREE
○ SUPER QUICK

⅔ cup Pork Rind "Bread" Crumbs (page 249)

1 tablespoon dried parsley

1 cup shredded Cheddar cheese

Nonstick cooking spray

1. Preheat the oven to 400°F.

2. In a medium bowl, combine the pork rinds and parsley.

3. In the food processor, pulse the cheese into a fine consistency. Add the cheese to the pork rind mixture and mix well.

4. Spray a muffin tin with cooking spray and add a thin layer of the pork rind and cheese mixture to the bottom of each muffin cup. Be careful not to pile them too high or they will not get crispy, and you want your chips crispy!

5. Bake for 10 minutes, until the edges are crisp. Let the chips cool for a few minutes and then transfer them to a plate. This mixture should make about 24 chips.

Variation: If you don't have a muffin tin, you can make circular mounds on a baking sheet.

MACRONUTRIENTS	67% FAT	32% PROTEIN	1% CARBS

PER SERVING (12 CHIPS): CALORIES: 315; TOTAL FAT: 24G; PROTEIN: 24G; TOTAL CARBS: 1G; FIBER: 0G; NET CARBS: 1G

BACON-WRAPPED CHEESE "FRIES"

PREP TIME: 15 MINUTES, PLUS TIME TO FREEZE **COOK TIME:** 15 MINUTES

Cheese wrapped in bacon? Yes, please! These are easy snacks or appetizers that will disappear from the plate as quickly as you can stack them up. *Serves 6*

○ COMFORT FOOD
● NUT-FREE

6 frozen full-fat mozzarella cheese sticks

Extra-virgin olive oil or ghee, for frying

12 bacon slices

1. Freeze the cheese sticks overnight.

2. In a skillet, heat ½ inch of olive oil.

3. Wrap each cheese stick with 2 bacon slices. Use 1 slice to pull around both ends of the cheese stick and then use the second slice to wrap tightly around the whole stick. Use a toothpick to secure the bacon.

4. Carefully add the cheese sticks to the hot oil.

5. Turn the sticks occasionally to get all sides of the bacon crispy.

6. Once crispy, place the bacon cheese sticks on a paper towel–lined plate.

Make Ahead: Place the cheese sticks in the freezer the night before; otherwise, they will just be globs of cheese with bacon on top (which I would totally eat, but that's not the desired outcome here).

MACRONUTRIENTS	70% FAT	28% PROTEIN	2% CARBS

CALORIES: 184; TOTAL FAT: 14G; PROTEIN: 12G; TOTAL CARBS: 1G; FIBER: 0G; NET CARBS: 1G

BACON-WRAPPED AVOCADO "FRIES"

PREP TIME: 10 MINUTES **COOK TIME:** 20 MINUTES

What is more keto than avocado wrapped with bacon?! These crispy-on-the-outside, smooth-on-the-inside snacks will have you addicted! Eat both servings for a meal, or split them into two servings for a yummy side dish. *Serves 2*

- ● ALLERGEN-FREE
- ○ COMFORT FOOD
- ◔ DAIRY-FREE
- ● NUT-FREE
- ● PALEO OR PALEO-FRIENDLY
- ○ SUPER QUICK

1 avocado, halved and pitted

1 teaspoon Chili-Lime Seasoning (page 244)

8 bacon slices

1. Preheat the oven to 400°F.

2. Slice the avocado into 8 wedges and peel off the skin.

3. Season the avocado with the chili-lime seasoning.

4. Wrap 1 bacon slice around each avocado wedge. Use toothpicks to secure, and arrange them on a baking sheet.

5. Bake for 20 minutes, until the bacon is crispy.

Variation: You can dip the fries in ranch dressing or any creamy dip.

MACRONUTRIENTS	73% FAT	19% PROTEIN	8% CARBS

CALORIES: 286; TOTAL FAT: 24G; PROTEIN: 13G; TOTAL CARBS: 6G; FIBER: 5G; NET CARBS: 1G

BACON-WRAPPED PICKLE "FRIES"

PREP TIME: 10 MINUTES **COOK TIME:** 20 MINUTES

Do you like pickles and bacon on your burgers? Well this tastes like that, only better! I love making keto-friendly French fry replacements—as you can see from the Bacon-Wrapped Avocado "Fries" (page 228)—so pickles were just a natural progression. *Serves 2*

- ● ALLERGEN-FREE
- ○ COMFORT FOOD
- ◐ DAIRY-FREE
- ● NUT-FREE
- ● PALEO OR PALEO-FRIENDLY
- ○ SUPER QUICK

8 pickle spears

8 bacon slices

1. Preheat the oven to 400°F.

2. Wrap 1 bacon slice around each pickle spear. Use toothpicks to secure, and arrange them on a baking sheet.

3. Bake for 20 minutes, until the bacon is crispy.

Variation: I dip mine in blue cheese dressing or Sriracha mayonnaise.

MACRONUTRIENTS	64% FAT	28% PROTEIN	8% CARBS

CALORIES: 190; TOTAL FAT: 14G; PROTEIN: 13G; TOTAL CARBS: 4G; FIBER: 2G; NET CARBS: 2G

BACON JALAPEÑO CHEESE CRISPS

PREP TIME: 10 MINUTES **COOK TIME:** 10 MINUTES

Cheese crisps are so simple and so yummy. I can't believe I used to buy Parmesan crisps at the grocery store instead of just making them myself. Plus, when you make them yourself, you can add fun flavors like jalapeño peppers and bacon bits to take them over the top! *Serves 2*

○ COMFORT FOOD
● NUT-FREE
○ SUPER QUICK

1 bacon slice

½ cup grated Parmesan cheese

½ cup shredded Cheddar cheese

1 jalapeño pepper, very thinly sliced

1. In a large skillet, cook the bacon over medium-high heat for about 8 minutes, flipping once, until crispy. Transfer the bacon to a paper towel–lined plate to drain and cool, then crumble it.

2. Preheat the oven to 350°F. Line a baking sheet with parchment paper or a silicone baking mat.

3. In a small bowl, combine the Parmesan and Cheddar cheeses.

4. Add ¼-cup mounds of the cheese mixture to the prepared baking sheet, leaving plenty of space between them.

5. Add a thin slice of jalapeño pepper and a few bacon bits to each cheese mound.

6. Bake for about 7 minutes, until the edges are brown and the middles have fully melted.

7. Set the pan on a cooling rack, and let the cheese chips cool for 5 minutes. The chips will be floppy when they first come out of the oven but will crisp up as they cool.

Variation: These are incredible with guacamole or simply topped with a small dollop of Dairy-Free Avocado Crema (page 257).

MACRONUTRIENTS	66% FAT	31% PROTEIN	3% CARBS

CALORIES: 221; TOTAL FAT: 17G; PROTEIN: 16G; TOTAL CARBS: 2G; FIBER: 0G; NET CARBS: 2G

CHEESE-IT CRACKERS

PREP TIME: 15 MINUTES **COOK TIME:** 15 MINUTES

Miss those cheesy crackers you snacked on pre-keto? These will be your best friend! The dough is very similar to the one I use for the Pepperoni and Pepperoncini FatHead Pizza (page 162), but with sharp Cheddar mixed in and copycat Everything Bagel Seasoning (page 247) on top. These take a little work, but they're really delicious. *Serves 4*

○ **COMFORT FOOD**
○ **SUPER QUICK**

½ cup shredded sharp Cheddar cheese

½ cup shredded mozzarella cheese

½ tablespoon cream cheese

¼ cup almond flour

1 large egg, beaten

Nonstick cooking spray

2 tablespoons Everything Bagel Seasoning (page 247)

1. Preheat the oven to 425°F.

2. In a microwave-safe bowl, add the Cheddar, mozzarella, and cream cheese. Microwave on high for 30 seconds. Stir and microwave again for 30 seconds, until melted.

3. In a mixing bowl, add the almond flour and beaten egg and mix well. Add the melted cheeses and mix well. Form the dough into a mound.

4. Spray two pieces of parchment paper with cooking spray and place the dough between the sprayed sides.

5. Using a rolling pin, roll the dough into a flat, thin, even layer. We're making crackers, so you want it pretty thin, about ¼ inch thick.

6. Once the dough is even, remove the top piece of parchment and slide the bottom piece of parchment and the dough onto a baking sheet.

7. Using a pizza cutter, cut the crackers into even squares. Sprinkle with the everything bagel seasoning.

8. Bake the crackers for 7 minutes and, using a spatula, flip the crackers. If you need to recut some of them, you can do so now.

9. Bake the crackers for 5 more minutes.

10. Cool for 10 minutes before serving.

MACRONUTRIENTS	70% FAT	28% PROTEIN	2% CARBS

CALORIES: 132; TOTAL FAT: 10G; PROTEIN: 9G; TOTAL CARBS: 1G; FIBER: 0G; NET CARBS: 1G

CHEESELESS ROASTED CAULIFLOWER NACHOS

PREP TIME: 10 MINUTES **COOK TIME:** 25 MINUTES

I probably couldn't do keto without cauliflower. It is so versatile and inspires so many different ideas, like these cauliflower nachos! The crispy roasted cauliflower is the perfect base for a whole variety of ingredients you can put on top. *Serves 2*

- ● ALLERGEN-FREE
- ○ COMFORT FOOD
- ○ DAIRY-FREE
- ● NUT-FREE
- ● PALEO OR PALEO-FRIENDLY

1 cauliflower head, cut into florets

2 tablespoons extra-virgin olive oil

2 tablespoons Chili-Lime Seasoning (page 244)

½ cup Dairy-Free Avocado Crema (page 257)

¼ cup Pico de Gallo (page 250)

2 jalapeño peppers, sliced

1. Preheat the oven to 400°F. Line a baking sheet with parchment paper or a silicone baking mat.

2. On the prepared baking sheet, arrange the cauliflower in a single layer and drizzle with the olive oil. Season with the chili-lime seasoning.

3. Roast the cauliflower for 25 minutes, stirring halfway through.

4. Transfer the cauliflower to a serving dish or large plate.

5. Spoon or pipe the avocado crema over the top of the cauliflower, and top with the pico de gallo and jalapeños.

Variation: This recipe is dairy-free, but if you want cheese, you can top the roasted cauliflower with shredded cheese and place back in the oven for 5 minutes.

MACRONUTRIENTS	75% FAT	6% PROTEIN	19% CARBS

CALORIES: 288; TOTAL FAT: 24G; PROTEIN: 4G; TOTAL CARBS: 14G; FIBER: 7G; NET CARBS: 7G

SALMON AVOCADO BOATS

PREP TIME: 5 MINUTES

If you are looking for a recipe that doesn't require any cooking at all, then you have found it. Smoked salmon and avocado are a delicious combination, and here you are just chopping both up with a few other ingredients and putting them back in the halved avocado skin as bowls! *Serves 2*

○ COMFORT FOOD
◐ DAIRY-FREE
● NUT-FREE
● PALEO OR PALEO-FRIENDLY
○ SUPER QUICK

1 avocado, halved and pitted

2 ounces smoked salmon, chopped

½ cucumber, diced (or 1 small Persian cucumber)

1 tablespoon finely diced red onion

1 tablespoon avocado oil mayonnaise

1 tablespoon Sriracha (optional)

Salt

Freshly ground black pepper

1 teaspoon fresh dill

1. Using a spoon, scrape out the avocado flesh and dice it. Keep the two halves of the avocado skin intact, as they will be the bowls.

2. In a mixing bowl, combine the salmon, cucumber, red onion, mayonnaise, and Sriracha (if using). Season with salt and pepper.

3. Spoon the diced avocado back into the avocado skins and add the salmon mixture. Top with the dill.

Variation: Use cream cheese or sour cream instead of mayonnaise if you eat full-fat dairy.

MACRONUTRIENTS	64% FAT	15% PROTEIN	21% CARBS

CALORIES: 188; TOTAL FAT: 14G; PROTEIN: 7G; TOTAL CARBS: 11G; FIBER: 5G; NET CARBS: 6G

REUBEN WRAPS

PREP TIME: 15 MINUTES

If you get a craving for a Reuben sandwich, this should hit the spot. All the same flavors, minus the Thousand Island dressing, wrapped up in the corned beef with a big, flavorful pickle spear in the middle. *Serves 2*

○ COMFORT FOOD
● NUT-FREE
○ SUPER QUICK

2 tablespoons avocado oil mayonnaise

1 teaspoon Worcestershire sauce

8 thin slices corned beef

4 slices Swiss cheese

4 pickle spears

1. In a small bowl, mix the mayonnaise and the Worcestershire sauce.

2. On a work surface, lay 2 overlapping slices of corned beef. Spread one-quarter of the mayonnaise mixture onto the corned beef, add a slice of cheese in the middle, and then the pickle spear at one end.

3. Wrap, starting on the pickle side, until the pickle is tightly wrapped in the center. Repeat three times to make four roll-ups.

Variation: If you can't imagine life without Thousand Island dressing, you can add 1 teaspoon of sugar-free ketchup to the mayonnaise mixture.

MACRONUTRIENTS	66% FAT	27% PROTEIN	7% CARBS

CALORIES: 491; TOTAL FAT: 36G; PROTEIN: 31G; TOTAL CARBS: 9G; FIBER: 1G; NET CARBS: 8G

DAIRY-FREE BUFFALO CHICKEN DIP

PREP TIME: 10 MINUTES **COOK TIME:** 3 HOURS

I have a recipe for Buffalo Chicken Dip in my last book, but it is full of dairy, so I thought I would make a version for my dairy-free friends! Use any leftover chicken that you have on hand for this recipe or try it with the Shredded Garlic-Lime Chicken (page 153). *Serves 2*

● ALLERGEN-FREE
○ COMFORT FOOD
◐ DAIRY-FREE
● NUT-FREE
● PALEO OR PALEO-FRIENDLY

½ teaspoon onion powder

½ teaspoon dried parsley

½ teaspoon garlic powder

Salt

Freshly ground black pepper

¼ cup avocado oil mayonnaise

1 teaspoon Dijon mustard

¼ cup buffalo wing sauce

2 cups shredded cooked chicken

2 tablespoons sliced scallions, green parts only

1. Preheat the slow cooker on low.

2. In a small bowl, mix the onion powder, parsley, and garlic powder, and season with salt and pepper.

3. In another small bowl, mix the mayonnaise, Dijon, and buffalo wing sauce.

4. In the slow cooker, arrange the chicken and sprinkle with the dry seasonings. Add the mayonnaise mixture on top.

5. Cover and cook for 3 hours.

6. Garnish with the scallions.

Variation: I like to serve this dip with veggies like celery, jicama, or cucumbers. I also love to dip my Pork Rind Chips (page 226) in it.

MACRONUTRIENTS	38% FAT	54% PROTEIN	8% CARBS

CALORIES: 348; TOTAL FAT: 15G; PROTEIN: 44G; TOTAL CARBS: 8G; FIBER: 0G; NET CARBS: 8G

ITALIAN WRAPS

PREP TIME: 15 MINUTES

Italian sandwiches are my favorite. I used to often crave a foot-long Italian sub. Luckily, I can get the same flavors in these easy wraps. The best part is the pop of flavor from the pepperoncini and the prosciutto that I add as my own take on an Italian sub. Look for high-quality, uncured deli meats. *Serves 2*

○ COMFORT FOOD
◐ DAIRY-FREE
● NUT-FREE
● PALEO OR PALEO-FRIENDLY
○ SUPER QUICK

4 thin slices salami

4 slices ham

4 slices mortadella

4 slices prosciutto

2 tablespoons avocado oil mayonnaise

¼ cup shredded romaine lettuce

4 whole pepperoncini peppers

1. On a work surface, layer the salami, ham, mortadella, and prosciutto, with the biggest slice on the bottom and the smallest slice on top.

2. Spread the mayonnaise on the stack of deli meat.

3. Add 1 tablespoon of shredded lettuce and 1 pepperoncini on top.

4. Roll tightly around the pepperoncini. Secure with a toothpick if needed. Repeat three more times with the remaining deli meat.

Make Ahead: Store in small ziptop bags for easy access throughout the week.

MACRONUTRIENTS	69% FAT	27% PROTEIN	4% CARBS

CALORIES: 402; TOTAL FAT: 30G; PROTEIN: 27G; TOTAL CARBS: 6G; FIBER: 2G; NET CARBS: 4G

PEPPERONI "TACOS"

PREP TIME: 10 MINUTES

I eat this snack more than any other. It could not be easier. In fact, I generally bring all three ingredients to the couch and just assemble them there in front of the TV. It's that simple but can be really delicious. I use marcona almonds that are marinated in olive oil and rosemary. *Serves 2*

○ COMFORT FOOD
○ SUPER QUICK

10 uncured pepperoni pieces

20 marcona almonds

2 tablespoons cream cheese, at room temperature

1. Spread equal amounts of cream cheese on each pepperoni piece.

2. Place 2 marcona almonds on top of the cream cheese, fold over the pepperoni, and eat like a mini taco. Repeat with the remaining pepperoni and almonds.

MACRONUTRIENTS	82% FAT	15% PROTEIN	3% CARBS

CALORIES: 262; TOTAL FAT: 23G; PROTEIN: 10G; TOTAL CARBS: 3G; FIBER: 1G; NET CARBS: 2G

SEAWEED SQUARE PILE UPS

PREP TIME: 10 MINUTES

I love salty seaweed snacks, and they make the perfect canvas to create quick sushi-inspired pile ups for a snack or fun appetizer. *Serves 2*

○ COMFORT FOOD

◐ DAIRY-FREE

● NUT-FREE

● PALEO OR PALEO-FRIENDLY

○ SUPER QUICK

6 seaweed snack squares

4 ounces smoked salmon

½ avocado, pitted

1 teaspoon soy sauce or coconut aminos

1 tablespoon Everything Bagel Seasoning (page 247)

1. On a work surface, lay out the seaweed snack squares in a single layer. Divide the salmon evenly between the seaweed squares.

2. Using a fork, scrape the flesh from the avocado, transfer to a small bowl, and mash. Mix in the soy sauce. Place a dollop of the avocado on top of each square. Sprinkle the everything bagel seasoning on top. To eat, fold like a taco and enjoy.

Variation: You can get really creative with the toppings on these. Imagine anything you find in sushi, like cucumbers and crab, and go from there.

MACRONUTRIENTS	45% FAT	40% PROTEIN	15% CARBS

CALORIES: 165; TOTAL FAT: 9G; PROTEIN: 19G; TOTAL CARBS: 6G; FIBER: 3G; NET CARBS: 3G

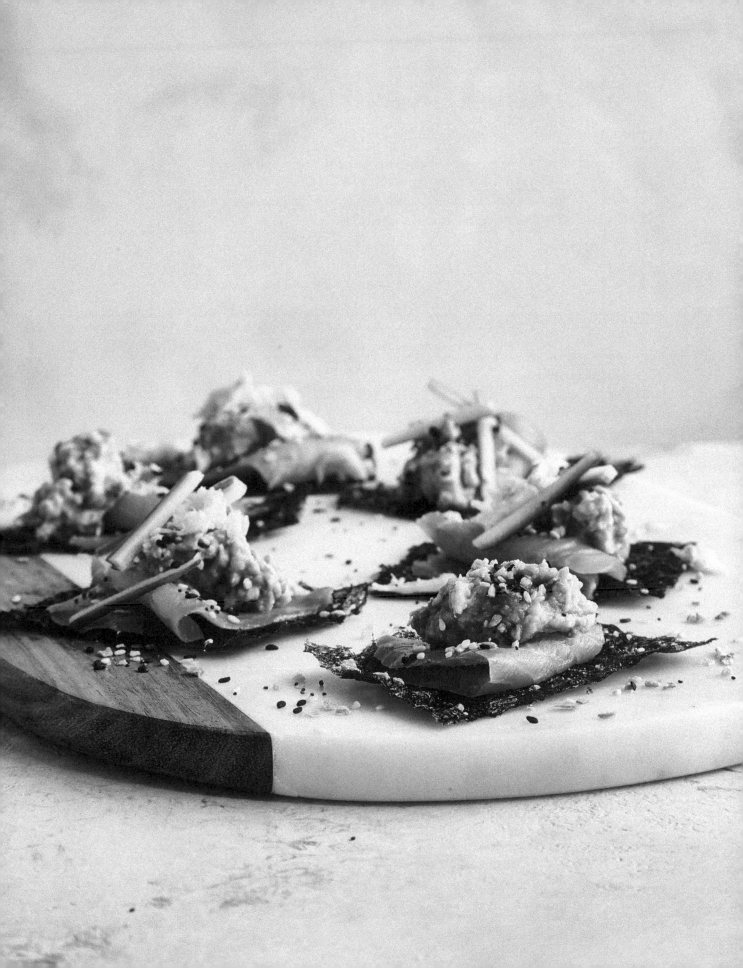

BACON AND AVOCADO CHEESE CUPS

PREP TIME: 15 MINUTES **COOK TIME:** 10 MINUTES

Cheese cups are so much fun and are delicious no matter what you fill them with, but BLTA (bacon, lettuce, tomato, avocado) is a hard combination to top! You are basically making larger-size cheese chips and then forming them into the shape of a bowl as they cool. *Serves 2*

○ COMFORT FOOD
○ SUPER QUICK

2 cups shredded Mexican blend cheese

¼ head romain lettuce, chopped

½ avocado, pitted, peeled, and diced

½ cup grape tomatoes, halved

6 cooked bacon slices, chopped

2 tablespoons sour cream

1. Preheat the oven to 350°F. Line a baking sheet with parchment paper or a silicone baking mat.

2. Add ½-cup mounds of shredded cheese to the prepared baking sheet and cook for about 7 minutes, until the edges are brown and the middle has fully melted. You want these slightly larger than a typical cheese chip.

3. Allow the cheese chips to cool for 2 minutes—they will be floppy when they first come out but will begin to crisp as they cool.

4. Before they are fully crisp, move each cheese chip into a muffin tin and form it around the shape of the cup to create a small bowl. The chip will fully harden in the muffin cup, which will make it really easy to fill!

5. Once the cheese cups have hardened, layer the romaine, avocado, tomatoes, bacon, and a small dollop of sour cream on each.

Make Ahead: The cheese cups store well in a sealed container for a few days.

MACRONUTRIENTS	71% FAT	24% PROTEIN	5% CARBS

CALORIES: 685; TOTAL FAT: 55G; PROTEIN: 39G; TOTAL CARBS: 9G; FIBER: 4G; NET CARBS: 5G

SPICY CRAB DIP

PREP TIME: 10 MINUTES **COOK TIME:** 40 MINUTES

Crab is one of my top-five favorite foods. I recently made this dip over the holidays for a party, and everyone devoured it. Serve this with veggie sticks or Pork Rind Chips (page 226), pipe it into hollowed-out cucumbers, or just eat it with a spoon because you can! *Serves 2*

○ COMFORT FOOD
● NUT-FREE

4 ounces lump crab meat

2 tablespoons cream cheese, at room temperature

1 tablespoon avocado oil mayonnaise

½ teaspoon freshly squeezed lemon juice

½ teaspoon Worcestershire sauce

¼ cup shredded pepper jack cheese

2 tablespoons grated Parmesan cheese

1 tablespoon sliced scallions, green parts only

½ teaspoon garlic powder

½ teaspoon hot sauce

Salt

Freshly ground black pepper

1. Preheat the oven to 325°F.

2. In a mixing bowl, combine the crab, cream cheese, mayonnaise, lemon juice, Worcestershire, pepper jack cheese, and Parmesan cheese. Mix well.

3. Add the scallions, garlic powder, and hot sauce, and season with salt and pepper.

4. Transfer the mixture to a small baking dish and bake for 40 minutes, or until it is golden and bubbly.

Make It Paleo: Use Dairy-Free Cream Cheese (page 258) and vegan Parmesan to make this paleo-friendly.

MACRONUTRIENTS	57% FAT	37% PROTEIN	6% CARBS

CALORIES: 221; TOTAL FAT: 14G; PROTEIN: 19G; TOTAL CARBS: 4G; FIBER: 0G; NET CARBS: 4G

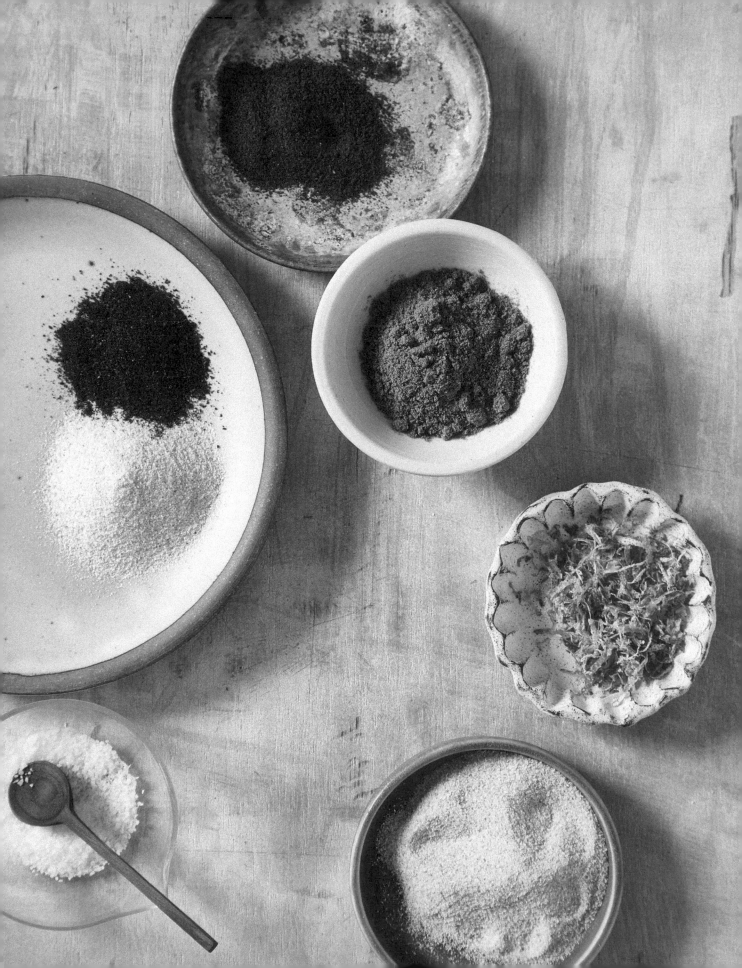

DRESSINGS, SAUCES, AND SEASONINGS

CHAPTER FOURTEEN

Opposite: Chili-Lime Seasoning

CHILI-LIME SEASONING

PREP TIME: 5 MINUTES

I LOVE chili-lime seasoning, and I use it a lot! If you asked my daughter, she would say I use it too much, but it is so good I can't help it. You can buy it premixed at the store, or you can make it yourself with spices you probably already have. *Serves 2*

- ● ALLERGEN-FREE
- ○ COMFORT FOOD
- ◔ DAIRY-FREE
- ● NUT-FREE
- ● PALEO OR PALEO-FRIENDLY
- ○ SUPER QUICK

1 tablespoon chili powder

1 teaspoon lime zest

½ teaspoon ground cumin

¼ teaspoon paprika

¼ teaspoon onion powder

¼ teaspoon garlic powder

Pinch salt

In a small bowl, mix the chili powder, lime zest, cumin, paprika, onion powder, garlic powder, and salt. You should end up with about 2 tablespoons of seasoning. You can keep extra in an airtight container or bag up to one week.

Variation: Add ½ teaspoon of cayenne pepper if you want it extra spicy.

| MACRONUTRIENTS | 39% FAT | 13% PROTEIN | 48% CARBS |

CALORIES: 16; TOTAL FAT: 1G; PROTEIN: 1G; TOTAL CARBS: 3G; FIBER: 1G; NET CARBS: 2G

TACO SEASONING

PREP TIME: 5 MINUTES

This taco seasoning is similar to the chili-lime combination but without the lime and with added oregano. Store-bought taco seasoning (also called Mexican seasoning) can be full of scary ingredients, so I like to make my own. *Serves 2*

● ALLERGEN-FREE
○ COMFORT FOOD
◐ DAIRY-FREE
● NUT-FREE
● PALEO OR PALEO-FRIENDLY
○ SUPER QUICK

1 tablespoon chili powder

½ teaspoon ground cumin

½ teaspoon dried oregano

¼ teaspoon paprika

¼ teaspoon onion powder

¼ teaspoon garlic powder

¼ teaspoon cayenne pepper

Pinch salt

In a small bowl, mix the chili powder, cumin, oregano, paprika, onion powder, garlic powder, cayenne pepper, and salt. It should make about 2 tablespoons of seasoning.

Make Ahead: If you use taco seasoning a lot, you can make a larger batch and store it for up to 6 months in an airtight container at room temperature.

MACRONUTRIENTS	36% FAT	16% PROTEIN	48% CARBS

CALORIES: 25; TOTAL FAT: 1G; PROTEIN: 1G; TOTAL CARBS: 3G; FIBER: 2G; NET CARBS: 1G

ITALIAN SEASONING

PREP TIME: 5 MINUTES

Italian seasoning is a classic. I love to add it to chicken dishes and really anywhere I want a savory touch. These are common seasonings, and you'll have the peace of mind of knowing exactly what is in your seasoning mix. *Serves 2*

● ALLERGEN-FREE
○ COMFORT FOOD
◐ DAIRY-FREE
● NUT-FREE
● PALEO OR PALEO-FRIENDLY
○ SUPER QUICK

2 teaspoons dried oregano

2 teaspoons dried basil

1 teaspoon garlic powder

1 teaspoon onion powder

1 teaspoon dried thyme

1 teaspoon dried rosemary

½ teaspoon red pepper flakes

Pinch salt

In a small bowl, mix the oregano, basil, garlic powder, onion powder, thyme, rosemary, red pepper flakes, and salt. It should make about 2 tablespoons of seasoning.

Variation: You can add 1 teaspoon of dried sage to the mixture if you have it on hand.

MACRONUTRIENTS	20% FAT	10% PROTEIN	70% CARBS

CALORIES: 23; TOTAL FAT: 0.5G; PROTEIN: 0.6G; TOTAL CARBS: 4G; FIBER: 1G; NET CARBS: 3G

EVERYTHING BAGEL SEASONING

PREP TIME: 5 MINUTES

This seasoning has gotten super popular. Some stores carry it, but it's not available everywhere, which is totally fine because you can make your own with just a few ingredients. If you are using the seasoning on something uncooked, such as in the Seaweed Square Pile Ups (page 238), then you want to toast the seasoning. But if you are using it on something cooked, like the FatHead Bagels (page 58), then you should sprinkle it on raw because it will toast when you bake it and you don't want to double toast it. *Serves 2*

● ALLERGEN-FREE
○ COMFORT FOOD
◐ DAIRY-FREE
● NUT-FREE
● PALEO OR PALEO-FRIENDLY
○ SUPER QUICK

2 teaspoons white and black sesame seeds

1 teaspoon poppy seeds

1 teaspoon onion powder

1 teaspoon garlic powder

1 teaspoon salt

1. In a small bowl, combine the sesame seeds, poppy seeds, onion powder, garlic powder, and salt.

2. To toast, in a dry skillet, add the seasoning mix over medium heat. Stir frequently and cook until the seasoning becomes fragrant and the sesame seeds are lightly toasted.

Variation: Flaked sea salt is a great replacement for regular sea salt in this recipe.

MACRONUTRIENTS	36% FAT	16% PROTEIN	48% CARBS

CALORIES: 25; TOTAL FAT: 1G; PROTEIN: 1G; TOTAL CARBS: 3G; FIBER: 1G; NET CARBS: 2G

RANCH SEASONING

PREP TIME: 5 MINUTES

When I first started cooking, I put dry ranch dressing mix on almost everything. It's super flavorful, and a little goes a long way. Luckily, it is easy to make yourself, which is awesome because then you know exactly what is in it. *Serves 2*

● ALLERGEN-FREE
○ COMFORT FOOD
● DAIRY-FREE
● NUT-FREE
● PALEO OR PALEO-FRIENDLY
○ SUPER QUICK

2 teaspoons dried parsley

1 teaspoon garlic powder

1 teaspoon onion powder

1 teaspoon dried dill

1 teaspoon dried mustard

1 teaspoon dried chives

Pinch salt

Pinch freshly ground black pepper

In a small bowl, combine the parsley, garlic powder, onion powder, dill, mustard, chives, salt, and pepper. Mix to combine. This recipe should make about 2 tablespoons of seasoning. Store any extra in an airtight container or bag for up to 1 week.

Variation: Add 1 teaspoon of onion flakes if you have them.

MACRONUTRIENTS	22% FAT	18% PROTEIN	60% CARBS

CALORIES: 20; TOTAL FAT: 0.5G; PROTEIN: 1G; TOTAL CARBS: 3G; FIBER: 1G; NET CARBS: 2G

PORK RIND "BREAD" CRUMBS

PREP TIME: 5 MINUTES

Using pork rinds in place of bread crumbs is one of my favorite keto tricks. All you need is pork rinds and a food processor. Whether it is for "breading" the outside of proteins or binding ingredients together, this will come in handy in your keto cooking adventures! *Serves 2*

- ● ALLERGEN-FREE
- ○ COMFORT FOOD
- ◑ DAIRY-FREE
- ● NUT-FREE
- ● PALEO OR PALEO-FRIENDLY
- ○ SUPER QUICK

½ cup crushed pork rinds

Pulse the pork rinds in a food processor until they resemble bread crumbs.

Variation: Parmesan cheese is a great addition, as are any variety of seasonings and dry herbs. You can also buy flavored pork rinds and grind them down to add instant seasoning to any dish.

MACRONUTRIENTS	44% FAT	32% PROTEIN	24% CARBS

CALORIES: 282; TOTAL FAT: 14G; PROTEIN: 22G; TOTAL CARBS: 17G; FIBER: 11G; NET CARBS: 6G

PICO DE GALLO

PREP TIME: 5 MINUTES

Pico de gallo is a super-easy, super-fresh salsa option. I love it on my Cheeseless Roasted Cauliflower Nachos (page 232), but you can also add it to eggs or any other dish where you want a pop of flavor. It really goes well with just about anything! I also like to mix it in when I make guacamole. *Serves 2*

- ● ALLERGEN-FREE
- ○ COMFORT FOOD
- ◐ DAIRY-FREE
- ● NUT-FREE
- ● PALEO OR PALEO-FRIENDLY
- ○ SUPER QUICK

1 small onion, finely diced

2 Roma tomatoes, finely diced

½ jalapeño pepper, finely diced (seeds optional)

½ cup chopped cilantro

1 tablespoon freshly squeezed lime juice

Salt

In a small bowl, toss the onion, tomatoes, jalapeño, cilantro, lime juice, and salt. Serve.

Variation: You can add minced garlic to the recipe too if you wish. Adjust the heat level to taste.

MACRONUTRIENTS	2% FAT	13% PROTEIN	85% CARBS

CALORIES: 32; TOTAL FAT: 0G; PROTEIN: 1G; TOTAL CARBS: 7G; FIBER: 2G; NET CARBS: 5G

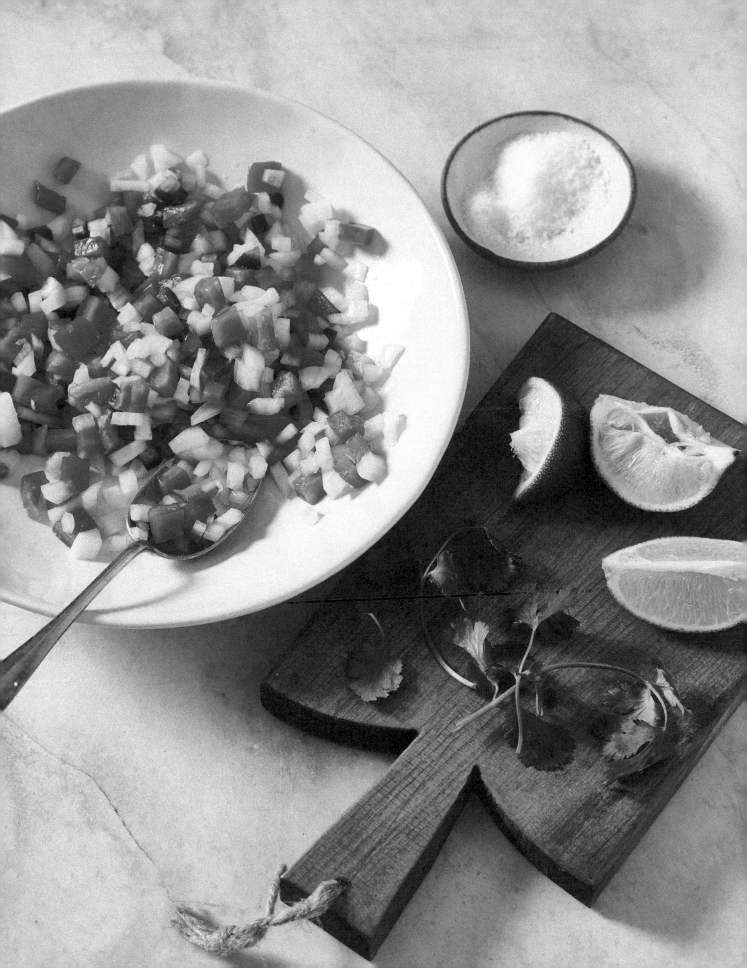

ENCHILADA SAUCE

PREP TIME: 5 MINUTES **COOK TIME:** 20 MINUTES

It is not easy to find gluten-free enchilada sauce, which is why this is a
nice alternative. Plus, you can be positive it has no added sugar in it. Just
keep in mind that the carb count in tomato products adds up quickly, so
be mindful of how much you use. *Serves 2*

- ● ALLERGEN-FREE
- ○ COMFORT FOOD
- ◔ DAIRY-FREE
- ● NUT-FREE
- ● PALEO OR PALEO-FRIENDLY
- ○ SUPER QUICK

5 ounces tomato purée

1 teaspoon garlic powder

1 teaspoon onion powder

1 teaspoon chili powder

½ teaspoon ground cumin

1 teaspoon hot sauce

1 tablespoon water

Salt

In a small saucepan, whisk together the tomato purée,
garlic powder, onion powder, chili powder, cumin,
hot sauce, and water. Season with salt. Simmer for
20 minutes, stirring occasionally.

Variation: You can add more hot sauce to taste. If the
sauce is too thick, add a bit more water.

MACRONUTRIENTS	17% FAT	13% PROTEIN	70% CARBS

CALORIES: 53; TOTAL FAT: 1G; PROTEIN: 2G; TOTAL CARBS: 9G; FIBER: 2G; NET CARBS: 7G

DAIRY-FREE TARTAR SAUCE

PREP TIME: 5 MINUTES

Tartar sauce is one of those things that I don't use very often, so I hate to buy a whole jar. Luckily, I usually have all the ingredients in my refrigerator anyway. Avocado oil mayonnaise is great because it is made with high-quality ingredients, whereas traditional mayo is usually made with subpar oils. *Serves 2*

- ● ALLERGEN-FREE
- ○ COMFORT FOOD
- ◐ DAIRY-FREE
- ● NUT-FREE
- ● PALEO OR PALEO-FRIENDLY
- ○ SUPER QUICK

¼ cup avocado oil mayonnaise

1 tablespoon chopped capers

1 teaspoon caper juice

1 pickle, diced

1 teaspoon freshly squeezed lemon juice

In a small bowl, combine the mayonnaise, capers, caper juice, pickle, and lemon juice. Mix well.

Variation: Some fresh dill is a nice addition if you have it on hand.

MACRONUTRIENTS	98% FAT	0% PROTEIN	2% CARBS

CALORIES: 184; TOTAL FAT: 20G; PROTEIN: 0G; TOTAL CARBS: 1G; FIBER: 0G; NET CARBS: 1G

WHIPPED CREAM

PREP TIME: 5 MINUTES

Homemade whipped cream is a million times better than the store-bought variety in my opinion, and since you're keto, you probably have heavy whipping cream in your refrigerator already. If you are dairy-free, check out the Dairy-Free Coconut Cream Whipped Cream (page 255) for your version. My mom always chilled the metal bowl in the freezer for 1 hour prior to making whipped cream, so now I do too. *Serves 4*

○ COMFORT FOOD
● NUT-FREE
○ SUPER QUICK

½ cup heavy whipping cream
½ teaspoon vanilla extract

1. In a chilled bowl, add the whipping cream and vanilla.

2. Using a hand mixer, mix on low until just combined, then switch to high for 2 minutes, until stiff peaks form.

Variation: I generally do not add erythritol to my whipped cream since I am usually adding it to something else that will have a sweet taste to it (on top of strawberries, for example). If you want extra sweetness, feel free to add it. I'd recommend 1 tablespoon of confectioners' erythritol.

MACRONUTRIENTS	93% FAT	4% PROTEIN	3% CARBS

CALORIES: 104; TOTAL FAT: 11G; PROTEIN: 1G; TOTAL CARBS: 1G; FIBER: 0G; NET CARBS: 1G

DAIRY-FREE COCONUT CREAM WHIPPED CREAM

PREP TIME: 10 MINUTES

I had never tried coconut milk before going keto, mainly because I hate coconut. Yup, I don't like the texture of shredded coconut, never have and never will, but funnily enough, it turns out I really do like coconut milk and coconut cream whipped cream! You must use chilled full-fat coconut milk, so place a can in the refrigerator the day before. As with traditional Whipped Cream (page 254), I like to chill the bowl for about an hour in the freezer before making this. *Serves 4*

- ● ALLERGEN-FREE
- ○ COMFORT FOOD
- ◐ DAIRY-FREE
- ● NUT-FREE
- ● PALEO OR PALEO-FRIENDLY
- ○ SUPER QUICK

1 (13.5-ounce) can unsweetened full-fat coconut milk

½ teaspoon vanilla extract

Without shaking the can, open it and add only the solid coconut cream to a chilled bowl. Add the vanilla and mix on high for 5 to 7 minutes, until stiff peaks form.

Make Ahead: You can store extra whipped cream in the refrigerator for up to 1 week, but it will harden up, so whip it up again with a whisk before eating.

MACRONUTRIENTS	92% FAT	3% PROTEIN	5% CARBS

CALORIES: 98; TOTAL FAT: 10G; PROTEIN: 1G; TOTAL CARBS: 2G; FIBER: 1G; NET CARBS: 1G

DAIRY-FREE HOLLANDAISE SAUCE

PREP TIME: 5 MINUTES **COOK TIME:** 10 MINUTES

Hollandaise sauce is one of those things that take a little patience to make, and patience is not one of my strong suits. But this dairy-free version is simple and can be made in a blender or with an immersion blender. The key to the sauce is the drizzling in of the ghee in step 3. Pour the ghee as slowly as possible to allow it to thicken properly, and your sauce is complete. *Serves 2*

○ COMFORT FOOD
◐ DAIRY-FREE
● NUT-FREE
● PALEO OR PALEO-FRIENDLY
○ SUPER QUICK

½ cup ghee

2 large eggs, yolks only

1 tablespoon freshly squeezed lemon juice

Dash hot sauce (optional)

Salt

1. In a small saucepan, add the ghee and melt over low heat.

2. In a blender, combine the egg yolks, lemon juice, and hot sauce (if using). Season with salt. Blend on the lowest speed for about 30 seconds.

3. With the blender still running on low, drizzle the ghee into the sauce through the feed tube as slowly as possible until it is all mixed in and thickened.

Make Ahead: Hollandaise will get hard in the refrigerator but will keep for a few days. Just reheat it low and slow on the stove top without boiling.

MACRONUTRIENTS	93% FAT	4% PROTEIN	3% CARBS

CALORIES: 281; TOTAL FAT: 29G; PROTEIN: 3G; TOTAL CARBS: 1G; FIBER: 0G; NET CARBS: 1G

DAIRY-FREE AVOCADO CREMA

PREP TIME: 5 MINUTES

Avocado crema can be made with sour cream, but this dairy-free version is made with full-fat coconut milk instead. Either way, it is delicious. I like to transfer the completed crema into a small resealable bag, cut a small corner off, and pipe it onto dishes. *Serves 2*

- ● ALLERGEN-FREE
- ○ COMFORT FOOD
- ◐ DAIRY-FREE
- ● NUT-FREE
- ● PALEO OR PALEO-FRIENDLY
- ○ SUPER QUICK

½ avocado, pitted and peeled

2 tablespoons unsweetened full-fat coconut milk

1 tablespoon extra-virgin olive oil or avocado oil, plus more if needed

1 tablespoon freshly squeezed lime juice

Salt

In a food processor, combine the avocado, coconut milk, olive oil, and lime juice. Season with salt and blend until smooth. If the consistency is thicker than you want, add a touch more olive oil or avocado oil.

Variation: You can add cayenne pepper or a dash of hot sauce if you want to add some spice.

MACRONUTRIENTS	85% FAT	3% PROTEIN	12% CARBS

CALORIES: 206; TOTAL FAT: 20G; PROTEIN: 2G; TOTAL CARBS: 7G; FIBER: 5G; NET CARBS: 2G

DAIRY-FREE CREAM CHEESE

PREP TIME: 5 MINUTES

Did you know you can make cream cheese with cashews? No? Me neither, until I started researching dairy-free life and discovered that it is possible to make a cream cheese–like mixture without dairy. It's pretty easy too—you just have to soak the cashews overnight, so plan ahead. *Serves 2*

○ COMFORT FOOD
◐ DAIRY-FREE
● PALEO OR PALEO-FRIENDLY
○ SUPER QUICK

½ cup raw cashews, soaked overnight in water and drained

2 teaspoons apple cider vinegar

2 teaspoons water

2 teaspoons unsweetened full-fat coconut milk

2 teaspoons freshly squeezed lemon juice

Salt

1. In a food processor or blender, add the cashews and process until they have a sand-like texture.

2. Add the vinegar, water, coconut milk, and lemon juice to the food processor. Season with salt and mix thoroughly for a few minutes, until the mixture resembles cream cheese.

Make Ahead: This recipe is for a small portion, so feel free to double it or triple it if you want to keep some around for the week. It can be stored in an airtight container for up to 7 days.

MACRONUTRIENTS	68% FAT	10% PROTEIN	22% CARBS

CALORIES: 241; TOTAL FAT: 20G; PROTEIN: 7G; TOTAL CARBS: 14G; FIBER: 1G; NET CARBS: 13G

DAIRY-FREE SOUR CREAM

PREP TIME: 5 MINUTES

Like the Dairy-Free Coconut Cream Whipped Cream (page 255), this recipe requires placing the can of full-fat coconut milk in the refrigerator overnight. This is what separates the cream from the liquid, and you only want the cream. Once you do that, this is very simple to pull together. *Serves 2*

- ● ALLERGEN-FREE
- ○ COMFORT FOOD
- ◐ DAIRY-FREE
- ● NUT-FREE
- ● PALEO OR PALEO-FRIENDLY
- ○ SUPER QUICK

1 (13.5-ounce) can unsweetened full-fat coconut milk

2 teaspoons freshly squeezed lemon juice

Salt

Without shaking the can, open it and add only the solid coconut cream to the food processor. Add the lemon juice and salt, and mix thoroughly. Store in an airtight container, refrigerated, for up to a week.

Variation: You can use apple cider vinegar if you don't have lemon juice.

MACRONUTRIENTS	88% FAT	4% PROTEIN	8% CARBS

CALORIES: 199; TOTAL FAT: 21G; PROTEIN: 2G; TOTAL CARBS: 4G; FIBER: 1G; NET CARBS: 3G

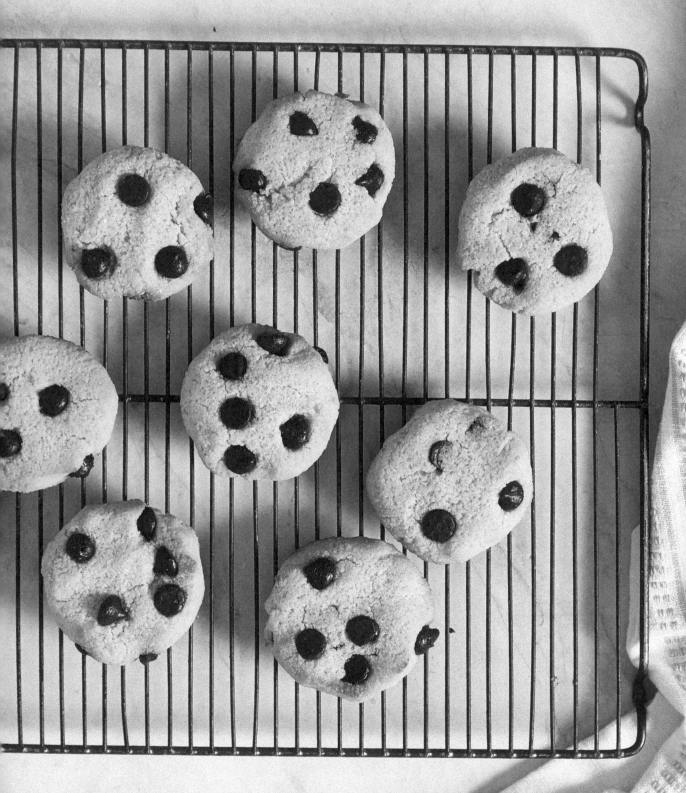

SWEETS

CHAPTER FIFTEEN

Opposite: Chewy Chocolate Chip Cookies

MACADAMIA NUT CLUSTERS

PREP TIME: 10 MINUTES, PLUS 10 MINUTES TO CHILL   **COOK TIME:** 1 MINUTE

I love macadamia nuts, and these are a keto-friendly version of the clusters they sell all over Hawaii. Whenever I eat them, I feel a little like I'm in a tropical paradise. You can use other varieties of nuts as well. *Serves 10*

○ **COMFORT FOOD**
○ **SUPER QUICK**

3 tablespoons butter

¼ cup heavy whipping cream

1 teaspoon vanilla extract

1 tablespoon erythritol

1 cup chopped macadamia nuts

¼ cup sugar-free chocolate chips

1. In a saucepan, melt the butter over medium heat. Stir continuously to brown, but do not burn. Once it reaches a golden color, remove from the heat.

2. Turn the heat down to the lowest setting and whisk in the heavy cream, vanilla, and erythritol.

3. Keep the mixture on the lowest heat and simmer for 5 minutes, whisking occasionally, until it thickens and darkens. Remove from the heat and stir in the macadamia nuts.

4. Line a baking sheet with parchment paper or a silicone baking mat.

5. Use a spoon to transfer 2- to 3-inch mounds of the mixture onto the baking sheet.

6. Chill the clusters for 10 minutes in the refrigerator.

7. In a small microwave-safe bowl, melt the chocolate in the microwave on medium power for about 30 seconds, depending on your microwave. Drizzle the melted chocolate over the chilled macadamia clusters and serve.

Variation: You can replace the macadamia nuts with pecans, walnuts, or any nut you choose. Additionally, if you are skipping dairy, you can use full-fat coconut cream instead of heavy whipping cream.

MACRONUTRIENTS	91% FAT	3% PROTEIN	6% CARBS

CALORIES: 162 ; TOTAL FAT: 17G ; PROTEIN: 2G ; TOTAL CARBS: 4G; FIBER: 2G ; NET CARBS: 2G; ERYTHRITOL: 1G

NO-BAKE LEMON BUTTER COOKIE BITES

PREP TIME: 10 MINUTES, PLUS 1 HOUR TO CHILL **COOK TIME:** 5 MINUTES

Does it get any easier than no-bake? These little bites will satisfy your sweet tooth and provide a simple base that you can add a lot of different flavors to. The lemon flavor is refreshing for those times when you want something sweet but aren't in the mood for chocolate. *Serves 10*

○ **COMFORT FOOD**

3 tablespoons butter

1¼ cups almond flour

2 tablespoons erythritol

1 teaspoon lemon zest

1 teaspoon vanilla extract

Pinch salt

1. In a saucepan, melt the butter over low heat.

2. In a small bowl, combine the butter, almond flour, erythritol, lemon zest, vanilla, and salt, and mix until fully combined. The mixture should be sticky like cookie dough.

3. Use a spoon to measure out 1- to 2-inch pieces and roll them into balls.

4. Place the cookie bites on a plate and refrigerate for about 1 hour.

Variation: You can get creative with the flavors in these cookie bites. I have replaced the vanilla and lemon zest with various flavor extracts, cinnamon, and sugar-free chocolate chips, and they are all delicious.

MACRONUTRIENTS	91% FAT	5% PROTEIN	4% CARBS

CALORIES: 53; TOTAL FAT: 5G; PROTEIN: 1G; TOTAL CARBS: 2G; FIBER: 1G; NET CARBS: 1G; ERYTHRITOL: 2G

GUMMIES

PREP TIME: 10 MINUTES PLUS 1 HOUR TO CHILL   **COOK TIME:** 5 MINUTES

Do you miss gummy bears? No need to! These gummies are delicious and easy to customize. You can leave out the heavy whipping cream, but it adds fat, making these mini fat bomb gummies. Grab your favorite silicone molds and get busy! Use any flavor of Jell-O to customize these to your taste. *Serves 4*

○ **COMFORT FOOD**

½ cup heavy whipping cream

1 (3-ounce) box sugar-free Jell-O, any flavor

1 tablespoon unflavored gelatin

1. In a small saucepan, heat the heavy cream over medium heat.

2. Add the Jell-O and gelatin, and stir until everything is combined.

3. Using a dropper, add the mixture to silicone molds.

4. Refrigerate for 1 hour to fully solidify. Unmold the gummies and transfer them to an airtight container. Store refrigerated.

Allergen Tip: You can use full-fat coconut milk instead of heavy whipping cream if you are not doing dairy. Place the can in the refrigerator the night before and only use the cream, not the liquid.

MACRONUTRIENTS	87% FAT	11% PROTEIN	2% CARBS

PER SERVING (6 GUMMIES): CALORIES: 114; TOTAL FAT: 11G; PROTEIN: 3G; TOTAL CARBS: 1G; FIBER: 0G; NET CARBS: 1G

CHOCOLATE-COVERED BACON

PREP TIME: 5 MINUTES, PLUS 30 MINUTES TO CHILL   **COOK TIME:** 10 MINUTES

Chocolate-covered bacon is the ultimate indulgence and quickly
became my favorite keto dessert the second I tried it! Sweet and
savory is the world's best combination, so it shouldn't be a surprise
that this is delicious. *Serves 2*

○ COMFORT FOOD
● NUT-FREE

8 bacon slices

4 ounces sugar-free keto-friendly
chocolate

1. In a large skillet, cook the bacon over medium-high heat
   for about 8 minutes, flipping once, until crispy. Transfer
   the bacon to a paper towel–lined plate to drain and cool.

2. In a microwave-safe bowl, melt the chocolate in 30-second
   intervals, stirring in between until smooth.

3. Arrange the bacon in a single layer on parchment paper
   and then pour the chocolate onto the bacon. I like to pour
   chocolate just on the top half of the bacon so that I can
   hold the piece by the bacon on the bottom when eating.

4. Place in the refrigerator to set the chocolate for about
   30 minutes.

Variation: One of my favorite ways to make this process even easier
is to use a ChocZero Dipping Cup per the instructions on the pack.
They come in white, milk, and dark chocolate, and harden quickly!

MACRONUTRIENTS	81% FAT	14% PROTEIN	5% CARBS

CALORIES: 454; TOTAL FAT: 43G; PROTEIN: 19G; TOTAL CARBS: 17G; FIBER: 9G; NET CARBS: 8G

CHEWY CHOCOLATE CHIP COOKIES

PREP TIME: 10 MINUTES **COOK TIME:** 15 MINUTES

I love puffy, chewy chocolate chip cookies, so these are my go-to keto replacement. I make these with sugar-free, keto-friendly chocolate chips. Nuts are also a great addition. The cream of tartar gives these cookies a great texture if you're like me and prefer soft cookies. *Serves 10*

○ COMFORT FOOD
○ SUPER QUICK

¼ cup unsalted butter

1¼ cups almond flour

¼ teaspoon salt

¼ cup erythritol

¼ teaspoon cream of tartar

1 large egg

1 teaspoon vanilla extract

¼ cup sugar-free chocolate chips

Make Ahead: These store very well in the refrigerator for a week. If you like nuts in your cookies, you can fold in macadamia nuts, pecans, walnuts, or any other chopped nut when you fold in the chocolate chips.

1. Preheat the oven to 350°F.

2. Line a baking sheet with parchment paper or a silicone baking mat and set aside.

3. In a saucepan or in the microwave, melt the butter. Place in a room-temperature container and let it set in the refrigerator for 10 minutes to cool down.

4. In a large bowl, combine the almond flour, salt, erythritol, and cream of tartar. Stir to combine.

5. In a small bowl, combine the egg, vanilla, and cooled butter. Whisk together.

6. Pour the wet ingredients into the dry ingredients and combine everything together with a large spoon or rubber scraper, then fold in the chocolate chips.

7. Scoop out 2- to 3-inch mounds of cookie dough and place on the prepared baking sheet. I like to flatten mine a bit.

8. Bake the cookies for 10 to 12 minutes, until the edges turn golden brown.

9. Let the cookies cool for 10 to 15 minutes before transferring them to a cooling rack to cool for an additional 15 minutes.

10. These will make puffy chocolate chip cookies with a chewy center. I absolutely love them cold, so I generally store them in the refrigerator.

MACRONUTRIENTS	83% FAT	7% PROTEIN	10% CARBS

CALORIES: 121; TOTAL FAT: 9G; PROTEIN: 2G; TOTAL CARBS: 3G; FIBER: 1G; NET CARBS: 2G; ERYTHRITOL: 5G

NUT BUTTER CHOCOLATE CHIP COOKIES

PREP TIME: 10 MINUTES **COOK TIME:** 12 MINUTES

These flourless cookies come together easily with your favorite flavor of nut butter. I use an almond and cashew mix, but you can experiment with other combinations. I like a nut butter that has a chunkier texture, which adds a nice bite to the cookies. *Serves 10*

○ COMFORT FOOD
○ SUPER QUICK

1 cup nut butter

1 large egg

½ cup erythritol

¼ cup sugar-free chocolate chips

1. Preheat the oven to 350°F.

2. Line a baking sheet with parchment paper or a silicone baking mat and set aside.

3. In a mixing bowl, combine the nut butter, egg, and erythritol. Mix with a stand mixer or hand mixer.

4. Fold in the chocolate chips.

5. Scoop out 2- to 3-inch balls of cookie dough and arrange on the baking sheet. I like to flatten mine a bit.

6. Bake the cookies for 10 to 12 minutes, until the edges turn golden brown.

7. Let the cookies cool for 10 to 15 minutes before transferring them to a cooling rack for an additional 15 minutes.

Variation: This recipe works great with low-sugar peanut butter.

MACRONUTRIENTS	78% FAT	9% PROTEIN	13% CARBS

CALORIES: 245; TOTAL FAT: 17G; PROTEIN: 5G; TOTAL CARBS: 8G; FIBER: 3G; NET CARBS: 5G; ERYTHRITOL: 10G

BLUEBERRY-LEMON CAKE

PREP TIME: 10 MINUTES **COOK TIME:** 20 MINUTES

I absolutely love blueberries, so this cake delights me. Plus, the lemon zest adds a wonderful freshness. This is a great dessert but also would be perfect for brunch. A few blueberries go a long way, so don't overdo it or the bottom of your cake will be mushy. *Serves 8*

○ COMFORT FOOD
● NUT-FREE
○ SUPER QUICK

Nonstick cooking spray

2 tablespoons butter, cut into 4 pieces, plus more if desired

4 large eggs

4 ounces cream cheese

¼ cup coconut flour

¼ cup erythritol

1½ teaspoons baking powder

1 teaspoon vanilla extract

1 tablespoon lemon zest

¼ cup blueberries, fresh or frozen

1. Preheat the oven to 425°F. Coat an 8-by-8-inch baking pan with cooking spray.

2. Put the 4 pieces of butter in the baking pan and place the pan in the oven for 2 to 3 minutes to melt the butter, but make sure it doesn't brown or burn. Remove from the oven.

3. In a food processor, mixer, or blender, process the eggs, cream cheese, coconut flour, erythritol, baking powder, vanilla, and lemon zest until thoroughly combined.

4. Pour the batter into the baking pan with the melted butter.

5. Drop the blueberries into the cake, evenly spreading them throughout.

6. Bake for 15 minutes, or until a toothpick inserted into the center comes out clean.

7. Serve warm and add more butter on top if you wish.

Make Ahead: Use a bundt cake pan with this recipe for a beautiful presentation. Sprinkle confectioners' erythritol on top for a final touch. This cake stores well in the refrigerator for a week.

MACRONUTRIENTS	72% FAT	14% PROTEIN	14% CARBS

CALORIES: 147; TOTAL FAT: 11G; PROTEIN: 5G; TOTAL CARBS: 5G; FIBER: 3G; NET CARBS: 2G; ERYTHRITOL: 2G

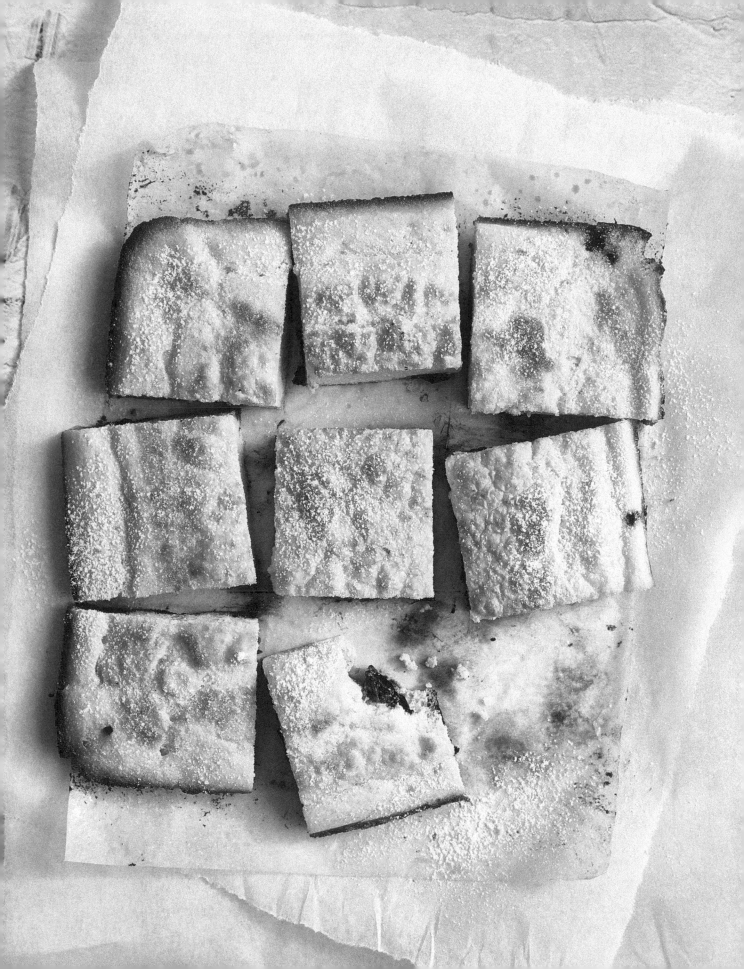

CHOCOLATE COOKIE BARK

PREP TIME: 10 MINUTES, PLUS 30 MINUTES TO CHILL   **COOK TIME:** 2 MINUTES

It is so easy to make chocolate bark, and you can add a whole assortment of things to your bark to make it unique. I like to make this after I've made a batch of Chewy Chocolate Chip Cookies (page 266) so I can crumble the cookies onto the bark. You can also use any other keto-friendly cookie. *Serves 10*

○ **COMFORT FOOD**

2 bacon slices

5 ounces sugar-free chocolate

1 keto-friendly cookie, crumbled

¼ cup chopped pecans

Pinch salt

1. In a large skillet, cook the bacon over medium-high heat for about 8 minutes, flipping once, until crispy. Transfer the bacon to a paper towel–lined plate to drain and cool, then crumble it.

2. Line a baking sheet with parchment paper or a silicone baking mat.

3. In a microwave-safe bowl, melt the chocolate in 30-second intervals, stirring in between until smooth.

4. Pour the melted chocolate onto the prepared baking sheet.

5. Sprinkle the crumbled cookie, bacon, and chopped pecans on top of the melted chocolate. Sprinkle with the salt.

6. Place in the refrigerator to set the chocolate for about 30 minutes.

7. Break the bark into 10 pieces and transfer to an airtight container. Store refrigerated.

Variation: Another great flavor combination is toasted, shredded coconut, slivered almonds, and salt.

MACRONUTRIENTS	70% FAT	12% PROTEIN	18% CARBS

CALORIES: 130; TOTAL FAT: 10G; PROTEIN: 4G; TOTAL CARBS: 6G; FIBER: 3G; NET CARBS: 3G

PECAN FAT BOMB

PREP TIME: 10 MINUTES, PLUS 30 MINUTES TO FREEZE **COOK TIME:** 5 MINUTES

These are the perfect bite when you need a little something between meals or a dose of healthy fats at the end of the day. Make an ice cube tray full and have them handy. *Serves 10*

○ COMFORT FOOD
◐ DAIRY-FREE
● PALEO OR PALEO-FRIENDLY

½ cup pecans

¼ cup coconut butter

¼ cup coconut oil

¼ cup ghee or butter

½ teaspoon vanilla extract

1 teaspoon pumpkin pie spice (optional)

⅓ cup erythritol (optional)

Pinch salt

1. Heat a dry skillet over medium heat. Add the pecans and toast, stirring constantly until slightly darkened.

2. Transfer the pecans to a cutting board and roughly chop.

3. Reduce the heat to low and place the skillet back on the burner. Add the coconut butter, coconut oil, and ghee. Heat until melted and then add the vanilla, pumpkin pie spice (if using), erythritol (if using), and salt.

4. Divide the chopped pecans into ice cube trays. Pour the coconut-ghee mixture over the pecans.

5. Freeze for 30 minutes, then unmold the bombs. Store in the freezer or refrigerator.

Variation: Adding 1 or 2 tablespoons of nut butter into these would also be tasty.

MACRONUTRIENTS	95% FAT	2% PROTEIN	3% CARBS

CALORIES: 181; TOTAL FAT: 19G; PROTEIN: 1G; TOTAL CARBS: 3G; FIBER: 2G; NET CARBS: 1G

SPICY CHOCOLATE FAT BOMB

PREP TIME: 5 MINUTES, PLUS 30 MINUTES TO FREEZE **COOK TIME:** 5 MINUTES

If you have never tried cayenne pepper with chocolate, you must! These sweet and spicy flavors make a great pairing. This version is a tasty fat bomb you can snack on whenever you need a little treat with a great dose of healthy fats. *Serves 10*

● ALLERGEN-FREE
○ COMFORT FOOD
● DAIRY-FREE
● NUT-FREE
● PALEO OR PALEO-FRIENDLY

¼ cup coconut butter

¼ cup coconut oil

¼ cup butter or ghee

2 tablespoons cacao powder

½ teaspoon vanilla extract

¼ teaspoon cayenne pepper

½ teaspoon ground cinnamon

2 tablespoons erythritol (optional)

Pinch salt

1. In a small skillet, melt the coconut butter, coconut oil, and butter over low heat. Once melted, add the cacao powder, vanilla, cayenne, cinnamon, erythritol (if using), and salt.

2. Pour the mixture into ice cube trays or silicone molds.

3. Freeze for 30 minutes, then unmold the bombs. Store in an airtight container in the freezer or refrigerator.

Variation: For a crunch, add chopped almonds, pili nuts, or macadamia nuts.

MACRONUTRIENTS	85% FAT	4% PROTEIN	11% CARBS

CALORIES: 190; TOTAL FAT: 18G; PROTEIN: 2G; TOTAL CARBS: 5G; FIBER: 3G; NET CARBS: 2G

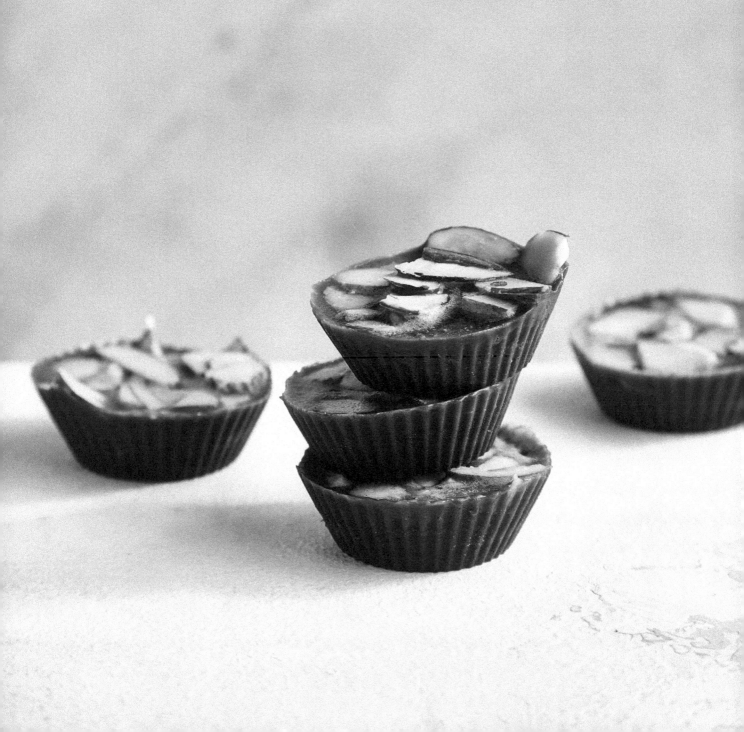

FATHEAD CINNAMON ROLLS

PREP TIME: 20 MINUTES **COOK TIME:** 20 MINUTES

FatHead dough can be used for so many things! I've shown you savory versions in chapters 4 and 10, but this is an unexpected sweet version. Mozzarella in cinnamon rolls?! It sounds weird, but just try it, and I promise you'd never know. *Serves 6*

○ **COMFORT FOOD**

FOR THE ROLLS

¾ cup shredded mozzarella cheese

2 tablespoons cream cheese

1 large egg

¾ cup almond flour, plus more as needed

Nonstick cooking spray

3 tablespoons butter or ghee

3 tablespoons erythritol

2 tablespoons ground cinnamon

FOR THE FROSTING

2 ounces cream cheese

1 teaspoon ground cinnamon

1 tablespoon heavy whipping cream

TO MAKE THE ROLLS

1. Preheat the oven to 400°F.

2. In a microwave-safe bowl, add the mozzarella and cream cheese, and microwave on high for 1 minute. Stir the mixture and microwave again for 30 more seconds, until melted.

3. Add the egg and almond flour to the cheese mixture and mix everything together gently. If the dough is sticky, sprinkle it with a little extra almond flour.

4. Spray two large pieces of parchment paper on one side with cooking spray and place the dough ball between the sprayed pieces.

5. Using a rolling pin, roll the dough into a rectangle that is about ½ to ¾ inch thick.

6. Peel off the top piece of parchment paper and place the dough and bottom piece of parchment onto a baking sheet.

MACRONUTRIENTS	77% FAT	10% PROTEIN	13% CARBS

CALORIES: 186; TOTAL FAT: 14G; PROTEIN: 4G; TOTAL CARBS: 6G; FIBER: 2G; NET CARBS: 4G; ERYTHRITOL: 5G

7. In a saucepan, melt the butter over low heat.

8. In a small bowl, mix the erythritol and cinnamon together.

9. Pour the melted butter over the dough, then sprinkle the cinnamon mixture on top. Roll into a tight jelly roll and then cut even rolls, about ½ inch thick. Arrange the cut rolls a couple of inches apart so they have room to expand on the baking sheet.

10. Bake for 10 to 15 minutes, or until golden brown.

TO MAKE THE FROSTING

In a small bowl or mixer, combine the cream cheese, cinnamon, and heavy cream. Using a knife, spread the frosting onto the warm rolls.

CHOCOLATE-AVOCADO MOUSSE

PREP TIME: 10 MINUTES

My favorite kind of dessert is the no-bake type that comes together in minutes! I crave this avocado and cacao combination. It is full of potassium and magnesium, so if your electrolytes are feeling a little out of whack, eat this for dessert or breakfast. Spinach may sound weird, but I promise you would never know it was in there. Be sure to put a can of coconut milk in the refrigerator to chill the night before and open it without shaking to easily separate the thick coconut cream. *Serves 2*

● ALLERGEN-FREE
○ COMFORT FOOD
◑ DAIRY-FREE
● NUT-FREE
● PALEO OR PALEO-FRIENDLY
○ SUPER QUICK

1 (13.5-ounce) can unsweetened full-fat coconut milk

1 avocado, pitted and peeled

3 tablespoons cacao powder

2 teaspoons vanilla extract

1 teaspoon ground cinnamon

2 tablespoons erythritol

1 cup fresh spinach (optional)

Pinch salt

Without shaking the can, open it and add only the solid coconut cream to the food processor or blender. Add the avocado, cacao powder, vanilla, cinnamon, erythritol, spinach (if using), and salt. Process until smooth and serve.

Variation: A kick of cayenne is great in here too if you like spice.

MACRONUTRIENTS	81% FAT	6% PROTEIN	13% CARBS

CALORIES: 539; TOTAL FAT: 51G; PROTEIN: 7G; TOTAL CARBS: 18G; FIBER: 12G; NET CARBS: 6G; ERYTHRITOL: 12G

BERRY-COCONUT CHIA PUDDING

PREP TIME: 10 MINUTES, PLUS OVERNIGHT TO SET **COOK TIME:** 15 MINUTES

Chia pudding is a delicious treat with tons of health benefits. This version is beautiful, with the blueberry purée and shredded coconut on top. These look super impressive and can be customized using the same coconut milk and chia base. To easily separate the coconut cream from the coconut milk, chill a can of coconut milk in the refrigerator the night before and open it without shaking. *Serves 4*

- ● ALLERGEN-FREE
- ○ COMFORT FOOD
- ◐ DAIRY-FREE
- ● PALEO OR PALEO-FRIENDLY

1 (13.5-ounce) can unsweetened full-fat coconut milk

1 tablespoon erythritol

1 teaspoon vanilla extract

¼ cup chia seeds

1 tablespoon blueberries

1 tablespoon raspberries

1 tablespoon diced strawberries

2 tablespoons sliced almonds

2 tablespoons shredded coconut

1. Without shaking the can, open it and add only the solid coconut cream to the food processor or blender. Process the coconut cream, erythritol, and vanilla until the mixture starts to thicken. Fold in the chia seeds.

2. In a small saucepan, add the blueberries, raspberries, and strawberries and simmer for 15 minutes. Mash them until smooth.

3. Pour half the coconut–chia seed mixture into four small glasses or bowls, then pour in the berry purée, then pour in the other half of the coconut–chia seed mixture. Cover the glasses or bowls and refrigerate overnight or for up to 3 days before serving.

4. Top with the sliced almonds and shredded coconut.

Variation: You can also use a frozen berry mixture instead of fresh berries.

MACRONUTRIENTS	79% FAT	7% PROTEIN	14% CARBS

CALORIES: 288; TOTAL FAT: 24G; PROTEIN: 4G; TOTAL CARBS: 11G; FIBER: 6G; NET CARBS: 5G; ERYTHRITOL: 3G

PEANUT BUTTER CUP CHIA PUDDING

PREP TIME: 10 MINUTES, PLUS OVERNIGHT TO SET

I love adding nut butter to my chia pudding for a quick and easy way to change the flavor and make it feel even more decadent. Topped with some cacao nibs or sugar-free chocolate chips, this dessert feels naughty even though it is full of nutritional benefits and quality fats. To easily separate the coconut cream from the coconut milk, chill a can of coconut milk in the refrigerator the night before and open it without shaking. *Serves 4*

○ **COMFORT FOOD**
◐ **DAIRY-FREE**
● **PALEO OR PALEO-FRIENDLY**

1 (13.5-ounce) can unsweetened full-fat coconut milk

2 tablespoons low-sugar nut butter or peanut butter

1 tablespoon erythritol

Pinch cinnamon

1 teaspoon vanilla extract

¼ cup chia seeds

1 tablespoon cacao nibs

1. Without shaking the can, open it and add only the solid coconut cream to the food processor or blender. Process the coconut cream, nut butter, erythritol, cinnamon, and vanilla until the mixture starts to thicken. Fold in the chia seeds.

2. Pour the mixture into four small glasses or bowls, cover, and refrigerate overnight or for up to 3 days before serving.

3. Top with the cacao nibs and serve.

Make Ahead: Any chia pudding lasts in the refrigerator for a few days, so you can make a few days' worth of breakfasts or desserts at once!

MACRONUTRIENTS	78% FAT	6% PROTEIN	16% CARBS

CALORIES: 350; TOTAL FAT: 30G; PROTEIN: 5G; TOTAL CARBS: 14G; FIBER: 7G; NET CARBS: 7G; ERYTHRITOL: 1G

CHOCOLATE CHIA PUDDING

PREP TIME: 10 MINUTES, PLUS OVERNIGHT TO SET

For many people chocolate is the holy grail of dessert foods. This chocolate treat uses cacao powder and mixes it with the creamy, fatty deliciousness of chia pudding. It doesn't taste healthy, but it is! To easily separate the coconut cream from the coconut milk, chill a can of coconut milk in the refrigerator and open it without shaking. *Serves 4*

- ● ALLERGEN-FREE
- ○ COMFORT FOOD
- ◐ DAIRY-FREE
- ● NUT-FREE
- ● PALEO OR PALEO-FRIENDLY

1 (13.5-ounce) can unsweetened full-fat coconut milk

3 tablespoons cacao powder

1 tablespoon erythritol

1 teaspoon vanilla extract

Pinch salt

¼ cup chia seeds

1 tablespoon cacao nibs

1. Without shaking the can, open it and add only the solid coconut cream to the food processor or blender. Process the coconut cream, cacao, erythritol, vanilla, and salt until the mixture starts to thicken. Fold in the chia seeds.

2. Pour the mixture into four small glasses or bowls, cover, and refrigerate overnight or for up to 3 days before serving.

3. Top with the cacao nibs and serve.

Variation: You can top this with Dairy-Free Coconut Cream Whipped Cream (page 255) to make it really feel like a dessert.

MACRONUTRIENTS	76% FAT	6% PROTEIN	18% CARBS

CALORIES: 314; TOTAL FAT: 26G; PROTEIN: 5G; TOTAL CARBS: 14G; FIBER: 8G; NET CARBS: 6G; ERYTHRITOL: 1G

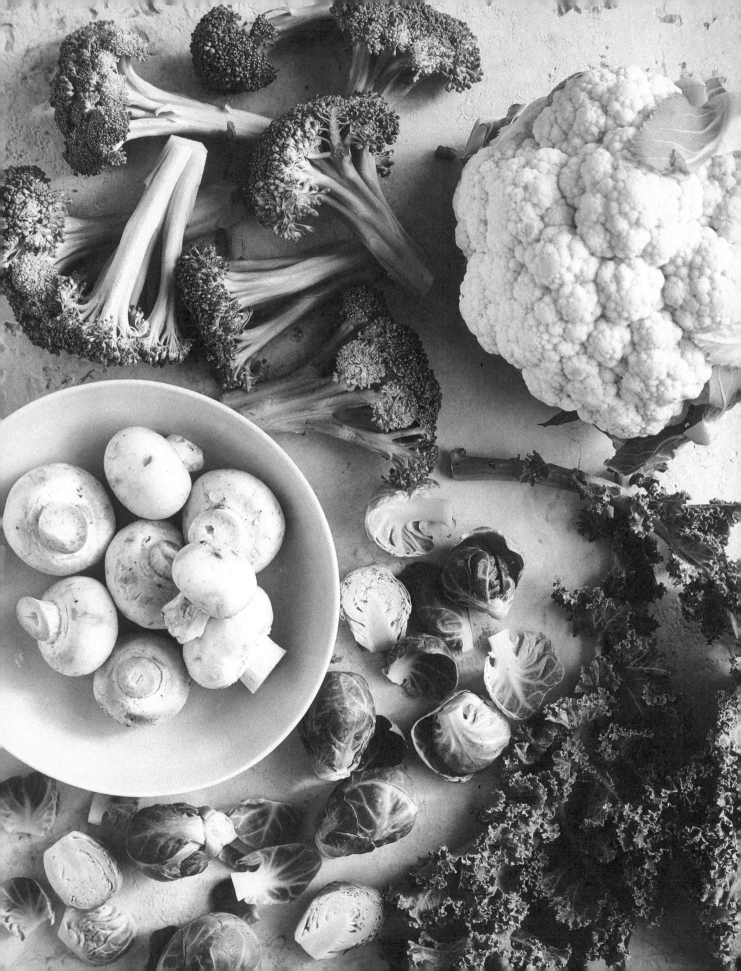

THE DIRTY DOZEN AND THE CLEAN FIFTEEN™

The Environmental Working Group (EWG) is a nonprofit, nonpartisan organization dedicated to protecting human health and the environment. Its mission is to empower people to live healthier lives in a healthier environment. This organization publishes an annual list of the twelve kinds of produce, in sequence, that have the highest amount of pesticide residue—the Dirty Dozen—as well as a list of the fifteen kinds of produce that have the least amount of pesticide residue—the Clean Fifteen. Please note that some of the foods listed here are not ideal for the keto diet (such as corn), but I'm presenting the EWG's list in its entirety.

The Dirty Dozen

The 2016 Dirty Dozen includes the following produce. These are considered among the year's most important produce to buy organic:

- Strawberries
- Apples
- Nectarines
- Peaches
- Celery
- Grapes
- Cherries
- Spinach
- Tomatoes
- Bell peppers
- Cherry tomatoes
- Cucumbers
- Kale/collard greens*
- Hot peppers*

The Dirty Dozen list contains two additional items—kale/collard greens and hot peppers—because they tend to contain trace levels of highly hazardous pesticides.

The Clean Fifteen

The least critical to buy organically are the Clean Fifteen. The following are on the 2016 list:

- Avocados
- Corn**
- Pineapples
- Cabbage
- Sweet peas
- Onions
- Asparagus
- Mangos
- Papayas
- Kiwi
- Eggplant
- Honeydew
- Grapefruit
- Cantaloupe
- Cauliflower

*** Some of the sweet corn sold in the United States is made from genetically engineered (GE) seed stock. Buy organic varieties of these crops to avoid GE produce.*

MEASUREMENT CONVERSIONS

VOLUME EQUIVALENTS (LIQUID)

STANDARD	US STANDARD (OUNCES)	METRIC (APPROXIMATE)
2 tablespoons	1 fl. oz.	30 mL
¼ cup	2 fl. oz.	60 mL
½ cup	4 fl. oz.	120 mL
1 cup	8 fl. oz.	240 mL
1½ cups	12 fl. oz.	355 mL
2 cups or 1 pint	16 fl. oz.	475 mL
4 cups or 1 quart	32 fl. oz.	1 L
1 gallon	128 fl. oz.	4 L

OVEN TEMPERATURES

FAHRENHEIT (F)	CELSIUS (C) (APPROXIMATE)
250°	120°
300°	150°
325°	165°
350°	180°
375°	190°
400°	200°
425°	220°
450°	230°

VOLUME EQUIVALENTS (DRY)

STANDARD	METRIC (APPROXIMATE)
⅛ teaspoon	0.5 mL
¼ teaspoon	1 mL
½ teaspoon	2 mL
¾ teaspoon	4 mL
1 teaspoon	5 mL
1 tablespoon	15 mL
¼ cup	59 mL
⅓ cup	79 mL
½ cup	118 mL
⅔ cup	156 mL
¾ cup	177 mL
1 cup	235 mL
2 cups or 1 pint	475 mL
3 cups	700 mL
4 cups or 1 quart	1 L

WEIGHT EQUIVALENTS

STANDARD	METRIC (APPROXIMATE)
½ ounce	15 g
1 ounce	30 g
2 ounces	60 g
4 ounces	115 g
8 ounces	225 g
12 ounces	340 g
16 ounces or 1 pound	455 g

RESOURCES

KetoInTheCity.com

This is my website, where I offer keto recipes, highlight my favorite keto products, and provide education on the ketogenic lifestyle.

Ruled.me and Ketogenic.com

These two sites are also great educational resources to learn about the science behind the ketogenic lifestyle. They are the two sites I visited the most when I first began my keto journey.

REFERENCES

American College of Allergy, Asthma & Immunology. "Tree Nut Allergy." Accessed May 15, 2018. https://acaai .org/allergies/types/food-allergies /types-food-allergy/tree-nut-allergy.

Asprey, Dave. "Bulletproof Intermittent Fasting: Lose Fat, Build Muscle, Stay Focused and Feel Great." *Bulletproof Blog*. Accessed May 15, 2018. https:// blog.bulletproof.com/bulletproof -fasting/.

Dr. Axe. "3 Macronutrients You Need and Top Food Sources." Accessed May 15, 2018. https://draxe.com /macronutrients/.

RECIPE INDEX

INDEX

ACKNOWLEDGMENTS

TO MY PARENTS I love you and thank you for always allowing me to believe I could truly do anything if I worked hard enough.

TO KAIA Having you as my daughter is my greatest joy. I love you to the moon and back, and I am so happy to always have you by my side.

TO MY FRIENDS AND FAMILY I am so inspired by my tribe, and I am so grateful to have such an amazing group of people around me. We are the people we surround ourselves with, and I am lucky to be surrounded by greatness.

TO THE KETO COMMUNITY I am so grateful to have found the passionate and supportive keto community on Instagram and online. You are an incredible group of people, each fighting different challenges but all trying to better yourselves. You all inspire me, and I hope I have been able to inspire you in return.

TO MY KITC TEAM Craig, thank you for helping me grow my passion for keto and food into so many wonderful opportunities. l can't wait to see what is in store for the future.

TO MY CALLISTO FAMILY Thank you so much for the guidance and support on both books. You welcomed me into the publishing world with open arms. I never imagined I would write a book, much less two. My first book's success is a testament to the amazing people at Callisto who led me every step of the way. To Elizabeth, Clara, Pippa, Eli, and the whole team, thank you for all the support.

ABOUT THE AUTHOR

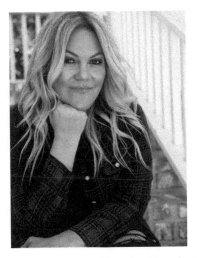

Jen Fisch, creator of the blog Keto In The City and Instagram account @KetoInTheCity_, is passionate about offering simple solutions for following the ketogenic lifestyle. She is a single, working mother who has battled autoimmune disorders for 20 years and has turned to the kitchen to find simple, delicious ways to make the ketogenic diet work for her busy lifestyle.

Jen is not a nutritionist or trained chef, just a determined mom who searched high and low for a way of eating that would reduce the inflammation caused by her autoimmune disorders and allow her to feel like the very best version of herself.

Her first book, *The Easy 5-Ingredient Ketogenic Diet Cookbook*, is an international best seller. The 130 recipes in the book were created to show people that keto can be delicious while also being simple to prepare. Jen believes in using easy-to-find ingredients to make eating keto as attainable as possible.

She lives with her daughter in Hermosa Beach, California.

DISCOVER MORE BEST SELLING
KETOGENIC DIET
TITLES FROM ROCKRIDGE PRESS

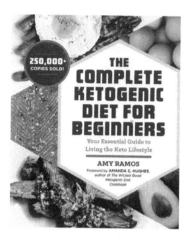

The Complete Ketogenic Diet for Beginners
Your Essential Guide to Living the Keto Lifestyle

Amy Ramos

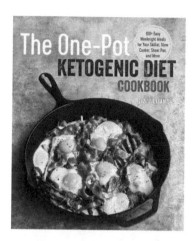

The One-Pot Ketogenic Diet Cookbook
100+ Easy Weeknight Meals for Your Skillet, Slow Cooker, Sheet Pan and More

Liz Williams

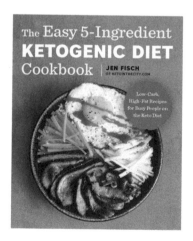

The Easy 5-Ingredient Ketogenic Diet Cookbook
Low-Carb, High-Fat Recipes for Busy People on the Keto Diet

Jen Fisch

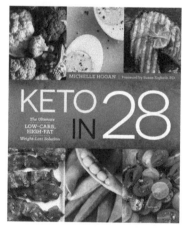

Keto in 28
The Ultimate Low-Carb, High-Fat Weight Loss Solution

Michelle Hogan

◪ ROCKRIDGE PRESS

Available wherever books and ebooks are sold